Contact!Unload

STUDIES IN CANADIAN MILITARY HISTORY
Series editor: Andrew Burtch, Canadian War Museum

The Canadian War Museum, Canada's national museum of military history, has a threefold mandate: to remember, to preserve, and to educate. Studies in Canadian Military History, published by UBC Press in association with the Museum, extends this mandate by presenting the best of contemporary scholarship to provide new insights into all aspects of Canadian military history, from earliest times to recent events. The work of a new generation of scholars is especially encouraged, and the books employ a variety of approaches – cultural, social, intellectual, economic, political, and comparative – to investigate gaps in the existing historiography. The books in the series feed immediately into future exhibitions, programs, and outreach efforts by the Canadian War Museum. A list of the titles in the series appears at the end of the book.

CANADIAN WAR MUSEUM
MUSÉE CANADIEN DE LA GUERRE

Contact!Unload
Military Veterans, Trauma, and
Research-Based Theatre

Edited by
George Belliveau and Graham W. Lea
with Marv Westwood

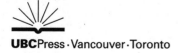

UBCPress · Vancouver · Toronto

© UBC Press 2020

All rights reserved. No part of this publication may be reproduced, stored in a retrieval system, or transmitted, in any form or by any means, without prior written permission of the publisher, or, in Canada, in the case of photocopying or other reprographic copying, a licence from Access Copyright, www.accesscopyright.ca.

29 28 27 26 25 24 23 22 21 20   5 4 3 2 1

Printed in Canada on FSC-certified ancient-forest-free paper (100% post-consumer recycled) that is processed chlorine- and acid-free.

Library and Archives Canada Cataloguing in Publication

Title: Contact!Unload : military veterans, trauma, and research-based theatre / edited by George Belliveau and Graham W. Lea ; with Marv Westwood.
Other titles: Container of (work): Contact!Unload (Play)
Names: Belliveau, George, editor. | Lea, Graham W., editor. | Westwood, Marv, editor.
Series: Studies in Canadian military history.
Description: Series statement: Studies in Canadian military history, ISSN (print) 1499-6251, ISSN (ebook) 1925-0312 | Includes bibliographical references and index.
Identifiers: Canadiana (print) 20200183990 | Canadiana (ebook) 20200184008 | ISBN 9780774862622 (hardcover) | ISBN 9780774862639 (softcover) | ISBN 9780774862646 (PDF) | ISBN 9780774862653 (EPUB) | ISBN 9780774862660 (Kindle)
Subjects: LCSH: Contact!Unload (Play) | LCSH: Psychic trauma – Alternative treatment – Case studies. |LCSH: Drama – Therapeutic use – Case studies. | LCSH: Veteran reintegration.
Classification: LCC PS8600.C663 C66 2020 | DDC C812/.6 – dc23

Canadä

UBC Press gratefully acknowledges the financial support for our publishing program of the Government of Canada (through the Canada Book Fund), the Canada Council for the Arts, and the British Columbia Arts Council.

This book has been published with the help of a grant from the Canadian Federation for the Humanities and Social Sciences, through the Awards to Scholarly Publications Program, using funds provided by the Social Sciences and Humanities Research Council of Canada.

Publication of this book has been financially supported by the Canadian War Museum.

Printed and bound in Canada by Friesens
Set in Helvetica Condensed, Myriad, and Minion by Artegraphica Design Co.
Copy editor: Frank Chow
Proofreader: Kristy Lynn Hankewitz
Indexer: Christine Jacobs
Cover designer: George Kirkpatrick

UBC Press
The University of British Columbia
2029 West Mall
Vancouver, BC V6T 1Z2
www.ubcpress.ca

To the men and women
who serve their countries,
past, present, and future,
and the loved ones who support them.

To Dr. Marv Westwood,
whose innovative work in group therapy
with veterans anchors this project,
and whose vision and passion fuelled it.

Contents

List of Illustrations / ix

Acknowledgments / xi

Letters of Appreciation / xii

Introduction / 3
Graham W. Lea and George Belliveau

Part 1: Researching, Developing, and Creating

1 Staging War: Historical Contexts of Theatre and Social Health
  Initiatives with Veterans / 21
  Michael Balfour

2 *Contact!Unload:* The Cauldron / 37
  Chuck MacKinnon

3 Facilitating Therapeutic Change through Theatre Performance / 38
  Alistair G. Gordon, Marv Westwood, and Carson A. Kivari

4 A Soldier's Tale: "Nobody Understood What I'd Done" / 46
  Britney Dennison

5 Listening through Stories: Insights into Writing *Contact!Unload* / 53
  Graham W. Lea

6 Suicides to Sydney / 65
  Foster Eastman

7 Coming Home / 71
  Tim Laidler

8 Reconnaissance and Reclamation: Learning to Talk about the War / 73
  Anna Keefe

9 Impact on Veteran Performers / 79
  George Belliveau, Blair McLean, and Christopher Cook

viii *Contents*

10 Holding on to the Script / 93
    Phillip Lopresti

CONTACT!UNLOAD: ANNOTATED PLAYSCRIPT / P1

Part 2: Performing, Witnessing, and Evaluating

11 Finding My Truth / 105
    Timothy Garthside

12 Unpacking *Contact!Unload* Using Relational-Cultural Theory / 109
    Candace Marshall with Graham W. Lea

13 *Contact!Unload* Revisited: Degrees of Separation / 123
    Lynn Fels

14 Remembering / 135
    Carl Leggo

15 A Poet(h)ic Reflection on *Contact!Unload:* Voices of Women
    through War / 139
    Heather Duff

16 Soldiers Lead the Way in the Fight for Mental Health among Men / 148
    John S. Ogrodniczuk

17 Audience Experience of Vicarious Witnessing in Performing War / 151
    Marion Porath, Marla Buchanan, and Elizabeth Banister

18 Understanding the Impacts of *Contact!Unload* for Audiences / 160
    Jennica Nichols, Susan M. Cox, and George Belliveau

19 Vulnerable Strength Seen / 172
    JS Valdez and Jennica Nichols

    Conclusion / 176
    George Belliveau and Graham W. Lea

    Contributors / 178

    Index / 184

Illustrations

1 HRH Prince Harry greets veterans after the performance of *Contact!Unload* at Canada House, London, November 2015 / 5

2 Five phases of therapeutic enactment / 9

3 Tableau / 11

4 Raising the Tribute Pole / 14

5 Tim Garthside sitting in front of the Tribute Pole with Chuck MacKinnon during a "Reach Out" moment / 62

6 lestweforgetCANADA mural / 66

7 Dale Hamilton carving the Tribute Pole / 67

8 The Tribute Pole in Canada House / 68

9 Panels from SERIOUSshit / 69

10 Marv Westwood and JS Valdez offering support to Tim Garthside during a rehearsal / 75

11 "It's like a fire team." Performing at Canada House / 87

12 Graham Lea setting up lights / P8

13 "There's too much ACTING" / P15

14 Marv Westwood as COUNSELLOR introduces the veterans / P16

15 "There'd be days of boredom" / P18

16 "A little white pill." Rehearsing Moment 10 / P34

17 "RAGE" / P41

18 Dale Hamilton showing Mike Waterman his "band of brothers" / P47

19 "Tight in the chest" / P53

20 Curtain call at Canada House, November 2015 / P61

21 Leaning over the body of a soldier / 127

22 Illuminating the military experience / 154

Acknowledgments

FIRST, WE WANT TO acknowledge Movember Canada for the initial funding for the *Contact!Unload* project through a grant guided by Dr. John Oliffe and Dr. John S. Ogrodniczuk.

We want to recognize the Faculty of Education at the University of British Columbia and Dean Blye Frank for ongoing support. Thank you to the Peter Wall Institute for Advanced Studies and the University of British Columbia's Office of the Vice-President of Research and Innovation for providing funding and support.

We are grateful to the Veterans Transition Network, whose team provided support at all stages of this project.

Foster Eastman and Tracy Averill have been ongoing champions of this project, providing studio space, countless hours, artistic contributions, and the care needed to have such a project succeed.

We are grateful to all the authors in this book for their valuable contributions and insights.

We also wish to thank the dozens of people who contributed in the creation of the various phases of this project: the counsellors who assisted; the artists, researchers, and audiences who witnessed the work; and the countless donors who offered financial and other supports that enabled the play to develop and travel across Canada and overseas.

Finally, and most importantly, we are so grateful to the veterans who shared and performed their stories: Chuck MacKinnon, Dale Hamilton, Warren Geraghty, Tim Garthside, Luke Bokenfohr, Stephen Clews, and Tim Laidler. We also appreciate the contributions of Phillip Lopresti, a tireless member of the *Contact!Unload* company, who was so inspired by the project that he enlisted in the armed forces. Thank you to these eight veterans for giving their energy and commitment to the project – you are the heart of *Contact!Unload.*

◇◇◇◇◇◇◇◇

I have watched the impact of *Contact!Unload* travel well beyond
the audiences that attended performances across Canada and
internationally. In sharing their own stories as part of their therapy, the team of artists and veterans, under the encouragement
and guidance of Marv Westwood and George Belliveau, spoke
a simple and direct truth that is still being passed by word of
mouth. Soldiers, their families, friends, and many other
Canadians continue to reliably hear the message that the com-
radeship that supported them in times of combat is still there to
support them in facing the anger, despair, and isolation that so
often accompanies mental injuries.

While there is still work to be done in destigmatizing mental
illness, the credibility given to *Contact!Unload* demonstrates the
effect it has had on the changing attitudes towards maintaining
and regaining mental health within the military community –
a success that any theatre company would be proud to claim as
their own – Bravo Zulu!

MATTHEW OVERTON, BRIGADIER-GENERAL (RETIRED)
MAY 30, 2018

◇◇◇◇◇◇◇◇◇

Marv Westwood and the passionate team of veterans, practitioners, and advocates that make up the Veterans Transition Network (VTN) are truly some of the pioneers of veteran wellness programming in Canada. Long before most Canadians had ever heard terms like "operational stress injury," this amazing group was revolutionizing peer-based therapy for injured veterans. What was developed from a simple idea out of the University of British Columbia two decades ago, has now grown to help veterans across Canada and around the world.

One of the amazing by-products of the "network" at the heart of VTN is the amazing army of veteran volunteers, donors, artists, and other passionate Canadians united in a desire to serve those who became injured serving us. I joined the VTN family in 2011 through my work on mental health with the True Patriot Love Foundation. In the years since, I have continued to praise, promote, and partner with VTN, both as Member of Parliament and as Minister of Veterans Affairs, because I know that their approach makes a real difference.

Contact!Unload grew out of the amazing work done by VTN. I have been fortunate to see this play performed on Parliament Hill and at the Invictus Games in Toronto. The play provides some powerful insights into the mental injuries that some of our veterans have to face, and the feeling of isolation that these injuries can cause. Performed by veterans themselves, it is a raw performance that draws people in and inspires those who are suffering in silence to get help.

Through its mental wellness programming, art therapy, and innovative theatre like Contact!Unload, the Veterans Transition Network is an innovator at breaking down the stigma associated with mental health and normalizing the conversation surrounding mental injuries from service. These conversations can empower someone who is suffering to "unload" some of the pent-up anguish and realize they are not alone on their journey back to wellness. Bravo Zulu to the VTN family. You are making a real difference in the lives of so many families.

HONORABLE ERIN O'TOOLE, MEMBER OF PARLIAMENT
JUNE 12, 2018

KENSINGTON PALACE

Received in the HC's Office

2 5 NOV 2015

HC — copy sent to Happe + one

17th November, 2015

Your Excellency,

I wanted to thank you for hosting me during my brief visit to Canada House on Remembrance Day last week.

I was delighted to find the opportunity to see the lestweforgetCANADA mural and to meet those involved in the CONTACT!unload production. Both pieces of work are extremely powerful in communicating the experiences of those on operations. Hopefully they will encourage others who are struggling to come to terms with these experienced to come forward and seek help.

I would be very grateful if you would please pass on my thanks to your team and to all those from the Veterans Transition Programme for making my visit possible, and to Marvin for the DVD which he kindly gave me. I much enjoyed meeting them all.

Best wishes and many thanks again.

Harry

His Excellency Mr. Gordon Campbell,
High Commissioner of Canada,
Canadian High Commission

Contact!Unload

Introduction

Graham W. Lea and George Belliveau

I'm a veteran. I served in Afghanistan in 2006. I don't know what to do anymore. I'm at the end of my rope. Nothing I'm doing is working. I'm thinking about killing myself. I don't know what to do. I need help. I don't need help tomorrow. I need help now.

– TIM GARTHSIDE[1]

THESE WORDS SHARED by Canadian Corporal Tim Garthside (Ret'd) vividly depict the urgent need for counselling resources for returning veterans. This book represents a call to action to responsibly address the sometimes difficult transition soldiers face when returning to civilian life. As of March 2018, 649,300 Canadian Forces veterans living today have served in foreign and domestic operations, including those in the Second World War, the Korean War, Cyprus, the Democratic Republic of the Congo, Somalia, and the former Yugoslavia, as well as conflicts in Afghanistan, Iraq, Libya, and Mali.[2] These numbers represent people whose lives were entwined with military service and therefore are at risk of suffering from mental health issues during training, active duty, and transition to civilian life. With support from a Movember Canada initiative on men's mental health, a team of counsellors, veterans, and artists from Vancouver, Canada, decided to tackle this issue using a creative approach.[3] In the winter of 2015, the diverse group consisting of military veterans, counselling psychologists, artists, and community members met to develop a theatre piece. They began a four-month experiment in blending theatre and therapy. This process led to the development of *Contact!Unload,* a fifty-minute play performed by veterans and community members.

The play, which can be found between Chapters 10 and 11, represents the heart of this book project, bringing to life the personal stories of veterans returning home from deployment overseas. The play was developed using a composite approach to research-based theatre in which military veterans (who had served in Afghanistan, Cyprus, and Rhodesia) participated with artists and clinicians in a series of artistic workshops that led to the production.[4] Through these workshops, the company explored the experiences of military veterans both in service and in their transitions to civilian life. This introductory chapter highlights the therapeutic and theatrical underpinnings of *Contact!Unload* and provides background on how the production evolved.

Contact!Unload emerged directly from the therapeutic work led by Dr. Marv Westwood at the University of British Columbia, where he co-developed the Veterans Transition Program (VTP) with Dr. David Kuhl. As of 2019, this highly successful group therapy program designed specifically for Canadian veterans has seen more than 1,000 returning military members participate. All eight military members from the *Contact!Unload* team have gone through the VTP, a central focus of which is therapeutic enactment (TE). The compelling stories of their transitions to civilian life and the hope offered through the VTP approach became the core content used to create the initial performance.

The play has since been adapted into a twenty-minute version that toured the United Kingdom in November 2015, and a thirty-five-minute version that toured Central Canada in 2016 and 2017. A professionally filmed version of the 2016 production is available online.[5] As of this writing, more than 3,500 people have seen the play across Canada and the United Kingdom, including federal policy makers and politicians at Parliament Hill in Ottawa, and HRH Prince Harry at Canada House in London (Figure 1). The most meaningful audiences have been fellow veterans as, at its core, the play is by veterans for veterans, sharing experiences of journeys home in body and spirit.

This edited book offers academic and artistic, personal, and theoretical perspectives from people directly involved in the performances of *Contact!Unload*, as well as those who witnessed the work as audience members. Through its polyphony of voices, it provides unique insights into this particular project, how the arts might help veterans work through and share their trauma, and the power of coming together to share expressions of humanity and hope.

Contextualizing *Contact!Unload*

Every day, an average of twenty-two veterans in the United States dies by suicide – nearly one life every hour of every day.[6] Such a devastating statistic demands continued development of interventions to address trauma-related stress injuries and facilitate veterans' transition home following their deployment. Innovative approaches for sharing these interventions with funders, researchers, and, most importantly, veterans must also be explored to broaden their exposure. As there are currently fewer military personnel being deployed from allied forces, more

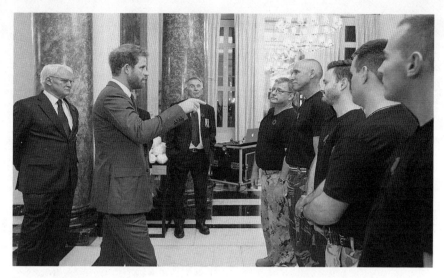

Figure 1 HRH Prince Harry greets veterans after the performance of *Contact!Unload* at Canada House, London, November 2015. Left to right: Gordon Campbell (Canadian High Commissioner to the United Kingdom), HRH Prince Harry, Marv Westwood, Chuck MacKinnon, Warren Geraghty, Mike Waterman, Luke Bokenfohr, and Stephen Clews | Photo by Frank Augstein/Pool via Reuters; used with permission.

attention has turned towards helping those who partook in those conflicts in their transition to civilian life. Bryan Doerries's work with his theatre company, Under the Wire, provides a compelling example of how theatre, in his case Ancient Greek plays, can produce a cathartic effect on serving and returning military veterans as well as their families.[7] Doerries engages professional actors to theatrically stage readings of Greek tragedies for military and veterans' groups across the United States and beyond, reaching thousands of military members and their families, along with health workers and the public. When veterans and civilians are brought together to listen to these tragic stories of mythical soldiers, important post-production conversations unfold, helping veterans and those close to them work through personal stories of struggle.

A number of other groups around the world are also using theatre to highlight challenges veterans face as they transition home following service. Similar to Doerries's initiative, these theatre efforts are aimed at listening to veterans' stories and stimulating post-production discussions with audiences. Rather than using professional actors, however, initiatives such as *Contact!Unload* and the selected companies we describe below feature veterans as the principal performers, who share their own personal stories of service.

The most expansive contemporary example is The Telling Project, based in the United States.[8] This countrywide initiative involves veterans publicly sharing their personal stories using a theatre-based approach. Founded in 2008, this not-for-profit initiative, spearheaded by Jonathan Wei with the support of Max Rayneard, has had a significant impact on both the performing veterans and the audiences they reach. Each production of The Telling Project is unique to the community where it is performed. The project's primary aim is to ease veterans' transition to civilian life, as Wei and other artists guide military veterans to tell their story of service along with their transition back to civilian life.[9] A director works with six to ten veterans from the community to develop theatre skills and use those skills to workshop and tell their stories for a minimum of five performances. In an interview with George Belliveau, Lisa Tricomi, a director and therapist who directed three Telling Project productions in Florida (Tampa, Orlando, and Pensacola), described the camaraderie and bonds developed during rehearsals and how these generate a forum of healing for the veterans.[10] Furthermore, as they share these stories with their local communities, the public is given an opportunity to deepen their understanding and appreciation of the emotional and psychological costs to those who serve in the military. As of early 2018, over seventy communities across the United States have engaged in The Telling Project, reaching thousands of audience members in more than seventeen states.

Stephan Wolfert, a medic and former infantry officer, developed DE-CRUIT, an initiative that also focuses on veterans sharing their stories.[11] His work aims to help veterans transition home while addressing the high post-traumatic stress (PTS) and suicide rates in the United States. Based in New York City, Wolfert invites veterans to participate in a drama-based process in which their personal writing is woven with Shakespearean text. The result is used as a stimulus to discuss their experiences of trauma as service members. Wolfert has teamed up with counselling psychologists at New York University to develop and evaluate this therapeutic model, and as of this writing they have worked with more than 500 veterans.[12] Wolfert also tours his one-man play *Cry Havoc!* which blends his personal experience of service with Shakespearean monologues, reaching veterans, health workers, and public audiences around the world.

The Feast of Crispian initiative also draws upon Shakespearean texts in its work with military veterans.[13] Based in Milwaukee, Wisconsin, this company has professional actors with military experience give workshops using Shakespearean text to help returning veterans in their transition. Led by therapists and actors, the company's goal is to work with veterans who are experiencing reintegration issues through modified acting exercises to help them get involved in theatre productions where they can once again feel part of a tightly knit unit of brothers and sisters. The stories of the participating veterans are woven into the Shakespearean texts as they perform the plays for a public that includes both military and civilians.

The Soldiers' Arts Academy, based in London, began much like the Feast of Crispian, as a veterans-based group performing Shakespeare's works for other veterans, their families, and the public, as a way for ex-servicemen and women to re-experience the camaraderie and bonds of their military service.[14] The group later partnered with other organizations to develop and write original plays. In 2012, in collaboration with Bravo 22 Company, it created the hugely successful play *The Two Worlds of Charlie F.*, written by Owen Sheers and directed by Stephen Rayne.[15] Based on interviews and workshops with military veterans, the play primarily features military personnel. It has evolved through more than 100 productions, including a 2014 tour to Toronto. The company has since developed another piece based on the lives of returning military veterans, *Soldier On*.[16] Written and directed by Jonathan Lewis, it vividly shows the impact of war on serving members and their families as well as the experience of veterans performing theatre. *Soldier On* has toured numerous cities in the United Kingdom with a cast of both veterans and professional actors. In addition to play creation and production, the Soldiers' Art Academy also has a mandate to deliver theatre workshops to schools, led largely by veterans. Engaging with theatre by performing and leading workshops has provided a place for veterans in the company to release some of their trauma and create new friendships and meaning in their lives.[17]

Re-Live, based in Cardiff, Wales, works in the field of arts and well-being.[18] In 2012, it partnered with local veterans to produce *Abandoned Brothers*. Led by artist and counsellor Alison O'Connor, the play uses narratives of veterans and visual art to share personal stories about the challenges of returning from war. The process of developing the play with veterans raised the question of how communities and countries support their servicemen and women psychologically and emotionally when they return home.[19] This same concern also arose during the creation of *The Return*, a theatre piece developed in Brisbane, Australia, in a partnership between local veterans and Griffith University (see Chapter 1).[20] Linda Hassall and Michael Balfour guided military veterans in co-creating a play about what it means to come home and the costs of serving one's country.[21] In both *Abandoned Brothers* and *Return*, Westwood's work on life review and therapeutic enactment are used by the facilitators to guide the veterans in the retelling of their stories and enhance the possibilities of therapeutic healing.[22]

Contact!Unload builds upon and complements these projects. Similar to a number of companies mentioned above, our Vancouver-based project makes use of a classical text to distance the trauma through poetic language, namely, Shakespeare's *Henry V*.[23] We found Shakespeare's poetic expression of human dilemmas and vulnerabilities generative when working with veterans. Furthermore, like many of the theatre projects discussed, *Contact!Unload* features veterans themselves onstage, sharing their personal stories in their own language. This creates a counterpoint to the Shakespearean language. The blending of personal and poetic texts is further complemented by the staging of a therapeutic enactment (see Moment 21 in the Annotated Playscript in this volume). This added feature makes *Contact!Unload* unique in that it incorporates the therapeutic model within the work, deliberately showing to the audience the process of working with soul injuries.[24] This creates an opportunity for audiences to "peek behind the therapeutic curtain," to vicariously witness what it is like for veterans to hold trauma in the body and, more importantly, possible pathways of releasing some of the burden of such traumatic injuries.

Veterans Transition Program and Therapeutic Enactment

The Veterans Transition Program is a residential group-based, veterans-only intervention intended to facilitate transition from active service to civilian life. The 100-hour program provides an environment of high-cohesion support by making the initial foci listening to each other's stories, seeing commonalities of experience among veterans who "have been there," and reinforcing the need to help one another. A key component of this support is paraprofessional soldiers, graduates of the VTP who have received additional VTP training. Within the group, there is a normalization of veterans' experiences, both in combat and in reintegrating into civilian life. Through teaching and practice sessions, veterans are given opportunities to develop knowledge of trauma, its symptom formation, and its impacts on the self and relationships. This is coupled with exposure to interpersonal communication strategies that help veterans develop skills for navigating important relationships and challenging interactions. As part of the program, veterans establish life goals to help guide them through personal and career development and growth. Family/spouse awareness sessions are also provided, recognizing that veterans' families also require support and growth to help facilitate the transition to civilian life.[25]

One of the central therapeutic interventions used in the VTP is therapeutic enactment (TE), an action-based group counselling strategy that asks participants to "enact critical events from their own life – [performing] the narrative,

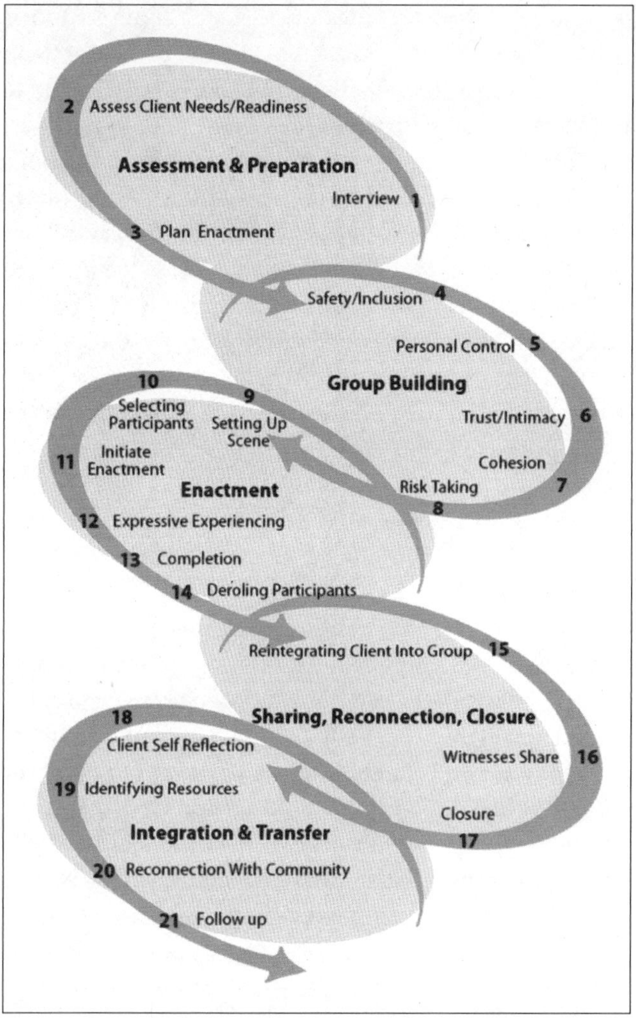

Assessment & Preparation

2 Assess Client Needs/Readiness

Interview 1

3 Plan Enactment

Safety/Inclusion 4

Personal Control 5

Group Building

10 9
Selecting Setting Up
Participants Scene Trust/Intimacy 6

11 Initiate
Enactment Cohesion

Enactment Risk Taking 7
8

12 Expressive Experiencing

13 Completion

14 Deroling Participants

Reintegrating Client Into Group 15

18 Sharing, Reconnection, Closure
Client Self Reflection
Witnesses Share 16

19 Identifying Resources

Closure
Integration & Transfer 17

20 Reconnection With Community

21 Follow up

Figure 2
Five phases of therapeutic enactment | From M.J. Westwood and P. Wilensky, *Therapeutic Enactment: Restoring Vitality through Trauma Repair in Groups* (Vancouver: Group Action Press, 2005), 8. Copyright 2005 by Marv Westwood and Patricia Wilensky; reprinted with permission.

going beyond language to express the self through action, movement, emotion, and reflection."[26] The five-phases of TE (see Figure 2) are designed to assist participants to integrate their trauma by guiding them through a "highly structured intervention in which [they] are able to externalize internal processes of trauma by enacting specific trauma narratives."[27] In the first phase, participants work with an experienced facilitator to assess their needs and readiness for the program and to design a plan. Central to this preparation is deciding upon the crucial life event that will be explored. With a clinical plan in place, the participant enters the group, which provides a space for building a safe and supportive environment. Once group trust is established, the participant and facilitator begin by walking within a circle of others, retelling the particular life event central to the participant's traumatization. After being familiarized with the story, fellow group members begin the enactment by taking on various identities in the story. Through techniques including role simulation, rehearsal, witnessing, and modelling, participants "access and express the buried feelings and negative cognitions attached to the problematic event."[28] Both the VTP and TE are inspired by arts-based therapeutic approaches that include the "protagonists, doubles, scenes, role playing, catharsis, and directors" of psychodrama.[29]

Following the enactment, those who took roles and those who witnessed are given an opportunity to provide feedback on how they were impacted. In the last phase of the TE process, participants are encouraged to look for ways of integrating the experience into achievable goals and objectives as they work on "dropping their baggage."[30] During a follow-up debriefing the day after the TE, the participant begins to reframe and consolidate the personal learning of the enactment.

Developing *Contact!Unload*

The development process began with Belliveau and Westwood bringing together a core artistic and research team in the fall of 2014, along with recruiting military veterans. During this time, Lea was brought into the project to develop the script as well as stage-manage and design the first production (see Chapter 5). During these meetings, preliminary framing structures for the play were discussed, including inspirations from the iconic St. Crispin's Day speech from *Henry V* and the metadramatic elements of Pirandello's *Six Characters in Search of an Author*.[31] Westwood drew upon his decades of therapeutic experience with veterans to suggest key themes to explore in the script, including:

- grieving: saying good-bye, letting another go
- giving back what was put on you
- taking back, claiming what was originally yours
- expressing your regrets
- saying you're sorry
- survivors' guilt.

These initial discussions were not intended to impose a structure on the final play but to provide a starting point for script development during the four-month development process with the veterans.

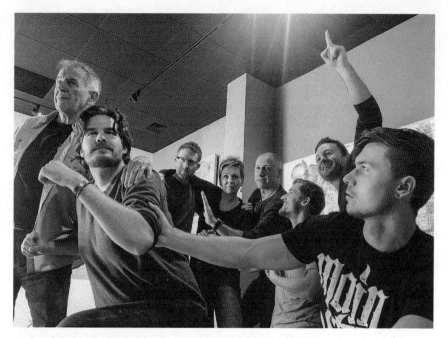

Figure 3 Tableau. Left to right: Marv Westwood, Dale Hamilton, Oliver Longman, Candace Marshall, Warren Geraghty, Tim Garthside, Mike Waterman, and Carson Kivari | Photo by Graham W. Lea; used with permission.

In January 2015, the core team began meeting with counsellors, community members, artists, researchers, and veterans in Foster Eastman's studio in Vancouver. This became our exploration space in which the artistic development team, guided by Belliveau, engaged in theatre-based approaches to elicit stories that were then woven into a research-based theatre script.[32] At the studio, rehearsals co-existed with the creation of the Tribute Pole, a companion visual art project by Eastman and the veterans memorializing Canadian troops killed in Afghanistan. This synergy between visual art and theatre was critical later in the project as the Tribute Pole became a centrepiece for the play (see Chapter 6). In this literal and metaphoric space of exploration, we engaged in a process in which information, primarily stories, was elicited from the veterans as key informants.

The development process frequently included sharing stories in a circle, building a sense of trust and community (see Chapter 12). One of the main features of TE is to *do* and, within the *doing*, discover, unpack, and process moments that might have been locked up or paralyzed. Building on this active component, Belliveau slowly introduced non-verbal drama-based activities to stimulate the veterans to express their stories through their bodies. One such activity was the creation of visual tableaux, frozen images (see Figure 3). After each activity, all participants joined in a circle with counsellors to debrief. Understandably, given the nature of the experiences involved, individuals would sometimes experience activation (triggering). Throughout all rehearsals and performances, counsellors were present who frequently provided individual or group debriefing when the need arose.

Initially, it was the veterans who would become emotionally activated from sharing and enacting their stories. As the process progressed, however, we came to realize that it was not only veterans who were experiencing emotional activation; many civilian members were similarly impacted, not just by the stories shared by the veterans but also by the space of deep personal introspection created as the veterans began allowing us into their realities. During this time, we became a company. In sharing and disclosing trauma-related stress injuries and vulnerabilities, the soldiers opened themselves up, sharing their experiences with the group. For our part as civilians, we were no longer only hearing but instead began to listen, understand, and feel the impact of the veterans' lived narratives.

Lea observed these exploratory sessions, generating observational notes as well as audio and video recordings (see Chapter 5). These data were complemented by previously published work about the veterans, interviews, video recordings, and Lea's own experiences. After two months of attending the weekly development sessions, Lea began writing the script with ongoing consultation from the group. Although it was not a verbatim script, many of the words in the play were uttered during the development sessions. Building on the work of Belliveau and Beare,[33] Lea held the stories, reshaped them, and moved them around, not to retell them exactly but to search for an essence of experience that might resonate deeply with theatrical audiences. Lea's close listening of the veterans' and the group discoveries in the development process resulted in a script the veterans saw as representative of their stories and experiences; as one of the veterans said, "You got it." It became clear to the theatre artists that this script could not have been created with the same degree of authenticity by analyzing collected research data. We needed to be in the space with the veterans, co-creating the work, experiencing the narratives with them – we needed to breathe the same air. The community experience that took place during the script development was critical as it generated ownership and elicited the unspoken kinship soldiers have with one another.

One of the challenges we encountered was the limited amount of time to elicit narratives, develop them into a script, and rehearse the script for public performance. While Lea and Belliveau had developed various productions using similar approaches, on this project we underestimated the impact of two constraints on the artistic development: the time required for veterans to buy into the project and trust the research team with their stories, and the time required for counsellors to guide veterans and other participants into, through, and out of the weekly development sessions (see Chapter 12).[34] As a result, we were not able to generate enough narrative material to develop a full script in time for performance. To address this, we incorporated some scenes from Linda Hassall's Australian play *The Return* into our theatre development. These scenes resonated deeply with our troupe, and with her permission, we adapted a few of her scenes into *Contact!Unload*.

The theatrical development process resulted in a 50-minute non-linear performance that fluidly moves through time and place to share five interweaving narratives:

1   The play opens with veterans performing a ceremonial raising of the Tribute Pole (see Figure 4). Once it has been raised, the character TIM sits under the pole, weighed down by the baggage he carries from his trauma-related stress injury (see Chapter 4).[35]
2   The narrative frame that structures most of the play is a rehearsal of the St. Crispin's Day speech from Shakespeare's *Henry V.* In the speech, HENRY speaks to his soldiers, who have already seen combat, as they prepare for a major battle. The director, unhappy with the actor's interpretation, brings in veterans to give the actor a sense of what it might be like to speak to people who have already experienced combat and what their reactions might be.
3   As the actor works on the speech, veterans are triggered by particular phrases. When this happens, they re-enact the traumatic memory.
4   After each flashback, a character tries to reach out to TIM, to help him find support to move through his injury. These attempts are brushed aside, until one veteran gives him a marching order to get help: "This is fucking enough" (see Moment 20).
5   The two then go to a session where Tim's TE is staged.

Two poems, written by the veterans, and songs were interwoven within the main script (see the Annotated Playscript in this volume). These interludes provided audiences with a respite from the intensity of the veteran's narratives.

With a draft script written, rehearsals began. During rehearsals, the focus shifted from generating content to refining and preparing for production, but the script continued to evolve, a process that continued through the various

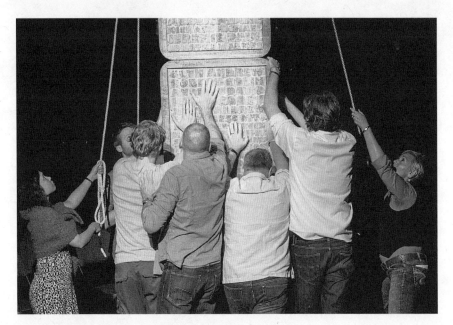

Figure 4 Raising the Tribute Pole. Left to right: JS Valdez, Oliver Longman, Tim Garthside, Warren Geraghty, Chuck MacKinnon, Dale Hamilton, and Candace Marshall | Photo by Blair McLean; used with permission.

iterations. The veterans took roles, playing themselves and supporting characters. Other community members and researchers took on supporting roles such as family and community members. During the pivotal TE scene, two founding members of the Veterans Transition Network (VTN),[36] Marv Westwood and David Kuhl, played themselves leading TIM through his TE. As such, they were able to provide immediate support for the actor or anyone else should they become activated while rehearsing or performing the scene (see Moment 21).

Sharing, rehearsing, and performing their narratives of trauma was challenging for the veterans. However, all of the original veterans continued to be involved in at least one further iteration of the project. Similar to Renée Emunah's description of the therapeutic potentials of self-revelatory performance, some veterans in our project described a sense of catharsis and normalization through telling their story over and over to a captive audience during rehearsals and performance (see Chapter 9).[37] Through the TE and the creation/performance of *Contact!Unload*, the veterans were given opportunities to control their narratives rather than have their narratives control them. While there were personal benefits for the veterans involved, one of the key reasons for pushing through the challenges and continuing with the project was to help other veterans, active service members, and their families to demystify and humanize trauma-related stress injuries.

Incorporating the arts into this research project also had direct impacts on audiences, the research team, and community members. Rather than being dispassionate observers, the researchers and community members were deeply embedded in the process (see Chapter 8). The space of vulnerability that emerged as the veterans began to share their stories created an opening for all team members to explore their own experiences and, following the veterans' lead, some members of the research team went through their own TEs. As a result of involvement in this project, several civilian members also made significant career shifts, with one of them entering the armed forces. The combined power of counselling psychology and theatre that structured this project enabled the veterans to continue their paths of recovery (see Chapters 2 and 11).

This book continues and extends the work of the *Contact!Unload* project, bringing narratives of veterans transitioning to civilian life to a larger audience. The authors share various experiences of *Contact!Unload* as members of the company, veterans, researchers, and audiences. The chapters are organized to tell a story of encountering, developing, performing, responding, and assessing the work. Anchoring the book is a full version of the script found after Chapter 10. The public performances and now this book have enabled the veterans' stories to reach families who had never heard the stories before, and other community members, including friends, researchers, counsellors, policy makers, and, most importantly, the veterans' "band of brothers (and sisters)" as we all try to understand what it means to come home fully.

Appendix: Production Timeline

Phase I

January–March 2015	Play development and rehearsals
April 30, May 1, 2, 2015	Studio 1398, Vancouver, BC

Phase II

November 4, 2015 (twice)	University of British Columbia, Vancouver, BC
November 8, 9, 11, 12, 2015	Canada House, London, UK
November 10, 2015	Central School of Speech and Drama, University of London, UK (abridged)
December 11, 12, 2015	Beatty Street Armoury, Vancouver, BC

Phase III

June 16, 2016	Staged reading, Foster Eastman's Studio, Vancouver, BC

September 15, 2016	BMO Goldcorp Theatre, Vancouver, BC
September 20, 2016	Royal Military College, Kingston, ON
September 21, 2016	Canadian War Museum, Ottawa, ON
September 21, 2016	Orange Gallery, Ottawa, ON
September 22, 2016	House of Commons, Ottawa, ON
September 22, 2016	Mill Street Brewery, Ottawa, ON (abridged)
May 5, 2017	Staged reading at University of British Columbia, Vancouver, BC

Phase IV

September 20 (twice), 21, 2017	Seaforth Armoury, Vancouver, BC
September 25, 2017	Canadian Institute for Military Health Research conference, Toronto, ON
September 26, 27, 2017	Invictus Games, Moss Park Armoury, Toronto, ON
September 28, 2017 (twice)	Invictus Games, Athletes' Village, Toronto, ON

Notes

This chapter is derived in part from Graham W. Lea, George Belliveau, and Marv Westwood, "Staging Therapeutic Enactment with Veterans in *Contact!Unload*," *Qualitative Research in Psychology* (February 22, 2018), https://doi.org/10.1080/14780887.2018.1442776.

1 Quoted in Chapter 4 of this volume.

2 "1.0 Demographics," Veterans Affairs Canada, March 27, 2019, https://www.veterans.gc.ca/eng/about-vac/news-media/facts-figures/1-0.

3 Men's Health Research (http://www.menshealthresearch.ubc.ca/projects), led by Drs. John Oliffe and John S. Ogrodniczuk at the University of British Columbia.

4 See G. Belliveau and G.W. Lea, eds., *Research-Based Theatre: An Artistic Methodology* (Bristol: Intellect, 2016); G.W. Lea, "Approaches to Developing Research-Based Theatre," *Youth Theatre Journal* 26, 1 (2012): 61–72, https://doi.org/10.1080/08929092.2012.678227. None of the veterans in this project served in the Second World War, but a recurring theme across a number of chapters in this book is connecting to the veterans of contemporary conflicts through narratives of veterans of historical wars such as the First and Second World Wars (see Chapters 8, 13, 14, 15, and 16). This is also noted by veterans (see Chapter 7) and in audience feedback (see Chapter 18).

5 "Contact!Unload," YouTube video of a performance at the University of British Columbia, September 15, 2016, posted by Peter Wall Institute for Advanced Studies, October 6, 2016, http://www.youtube.com/watch?v=Qjbfz_wReLI.

6 J. Kemp and R. Bossarte, *Suicide Data Report, 2012* (Washington, DC: Department of Veterans Affairs, 2012), http://www.va.gov/opa/docs/Suicide-Data-Report-2012-final.pdf. As of this writing, no public sources were available that accurately account for Canadian veterans dying by suicide.

7 B. Doerries, *The Theater of War: What Ancient Greek Tragedies Can Teach Us Today* (New York: Alfred A. Knopf, 2015).

8 http://thetellingproject.org.

9 M.L. Martinez, "Activism on Stage: The Telling Project: An Interview with Jon Wei, Founder and Director," *American Book Review* 34, 5 (2013): 8, https://doi.org/10.1353/abr.2013.0098.

10 L. Tricomi, personal communication with George Belliveau, February 27, 2018.

11 http://www.decruit.org.

12 A. Ali and S. Wolfert, "Theatre as a Treatment for Posttraumatic Stress in Military Veterans: Exploring the Psychotherapeutic Potential of Mimetic Induction," *The Arts in Psychotherapy* 50 (2016): 58–65, https://doi.org/10.1016/j.aip.2016.06.004.

13 http://www.feastofcrispian.org.

14 Its name changed in 2017 from the Combat Veteran Players. http://www.soldiersartsacademy.com.

15 O. Sheers, *The Two Worlds of Charlie F.* (London: Faber and Faber, 2012), http://www.charlie-f.com.

16 C. Hart, "Soldier On, Playground Theatre," *The Times* (UK), April 1, 2018, https://www.thetimes.co.uk/article/theatre-review-soldier-on-playground-theatre-tgcd27770.

17 M. Donnelly, "Can Shakespeare Heal? One Director's Quest to Help Treat PTSD," *Daily Signal*, September 7, 2015, http://dailysignal.com/2015/09/07/can-shakespeare-heal-one-directors-quest-to-help-treat-ptsd.

18 http://www.re-live.org.uk.

19 A. O'Connor, "Abandoned Brothers, Life Story Theatre with Veterans and Their Families," *Arts and Health* 7, 2 (2015): 151–60, https://doi.org/10.1080/17533015.2015.1011177. After the production of *Abandoned Brothers*, the veterans' group wished to remain connected, so it formed the Coming Home choir, which meets weekly.

20 L. Hassall, *The Return*, unpublished play, 2014.

21 L. Hassall and M. Balfour, "Transitioning Home: Research-Based Theatre with Returning Servicemen and Their Families," in *Research-Based Theatre: An Artistic Methodology*, ed. G. Belliveau and G.W. Lea, 103–16 (Bristol: Intellect, 2016).

22 M.J. Westwood, "The Veterans' Transition Program: Therapeutic Enactment in Action," *Educational Insights* 13, 2 (2009), http://einsights.ogpr.educ.ubc.ca/v13n02/articles/westwood/index.html.

23 B. Mowat, P. Werstine, M. Poston, and R. Niles, eds., *Henry V* (Washington, DC: Folger Shakespeare Library, n.d.), http://www.folgerdigitaltexts.org.

24 D.T. Lohrey, "Soul Death and the Legacy of Total War," *Perichoresis* 15, 2 (2017): 59–82, https://doi.org/10.1515/perc-2017-0010.

25 M.J. Westwood, H. McLean, D. Cave, W. Borgen, and P. Slakov, "Coming Home: A Group-Based Approach for Assisting Military Veterans in Transition," *Journal for Specialists in Group Work* 35, 1 (2010): 44–68, https://doi.org/10.1080/01933920903466059.

26 Westwood, "The Veterans' Transition Program," para. 1. Other interventions, such as narrative writing and verbal presentation, symptom identification, and rehearsal, are used as part of the VTP. However, the focus in this project was on TE.

27 Westwood et al., "Coming Home," 49.

28 Ibid., 49–50.

29 M.J. Westwood and P. Wilensky, *Therapeutic Enactment: Restoring Vitality through Trauma Repair in Groups* (Vancouver: Group Action Press, 2005), 2.

30 Westwood et al., "Coming Home," 49.

31 L. Pirandello, *Six Characters in Search of an Author* (London: Heinemann, 1954).

32 On theatre-based approaches, see G. Belliveau, "Using Drama to Build Community in Canadian Schools," in *Creating Together: An Interdisciplinary Workshop of Participatory Community-Based and Collaborative Arts Practices and Scholarship*, ed. A. Sinner and D. Conrad, 131–43 (Waterloo, ON: Wilfrid Laurier University Press, 2015); and J. Norris, *Playbuilding as Qualitative Research: A Participatory Arts-Based Approach* (Walnut Creek, CA: Left Coast, 2009). On developing research-based theatre scripts, see Belliveau and Lea, *Research-Based Theatre*; T. Goldstein, J. Gray, J. Salisbury, and P. Snell, "When

Qualitative Research Meets Theater: The Complexities of Performed Ethnography and Research-Informed Theater Project Design," *Qualitative Inquiry* 20, 5 (2014): 674–85, https://doi.org/10.1177/1077800413513738; and R. Sallis, "Ethnographic Performance: A Change Agent for Drama Teaching and Learning," *Research in Drama Education: The Journal of Applied Theatre and Performance* 19, 3 (2014): 313–25, https://doi.org/10.1080/13569783.2014.928011.

33 G. Belliveau and D. Beare, "Dialoguing Scripted Data," in *Being with A/r/tography*, ed. S. Springgay, R. Irwin, C. Leggo, and P. Gouzouasis, 141–52 (Rotterdam: Sense, 2008).

34 For examples of productions using similar approaches, see G. Belliveau, *"You Didn't Do Anything! A Research Play on Bullying," Educational Insights* 12, 2 (2008), http://www.ccfi.educ.ubc.ca/publication/insights/v12n02/articles/belliveau/index.html; A. Wager, G. Belliveau, J. Beck, snd G.W. Lea, " Exploring *Drama as an Additional Language* through Research-Based Theatre," *Scenario: Journal for Drama and Theatre in Foreign and Second Language Education* 3, 2 (2009), http://publish.ucc.ie/scenario/2009/02/wagerbelliveau/04/en; and G.W. Lea, "Homa Bay Memories: Using Research-Based Theatre to Explore a Narrative Inheritance" (PhD dissertation, University of British Columbia, 2013), https://open.library.ubc.ca/cIRcle/collections/24/items/1.0165696.

35 Veterans and civilians played themselves in the performance. Names in uppercase are character names. For example, Marv Westwood played the character MARV.

36 VTN is the organization that implements the Veterans Transition Program (VTP).

37 R. Emunah, "Self-Revelatory Performance: A Form of Drama Therapy and Theatre," *Drama Therapy Review* 1, 1 (2015): 71–85, https://doi.org/10.1386/dtr.1.1.71_1.

Part 1
Researching, Developing, and Creating

1

Staging War
Historical Contexts of Theatre and Social Health Initiatives with Veterans

Michael Balfour

> *These shattered men believe that they failed friends and neglected moral meaning when the chips were down, and they blame themselves. They are welded to their guilt using the remainder of their lives to expiate their past sins.*
>
> – THEODORE NADELSON[1]

IN THE LAST DECADE, thousands of military personnel from the United States, the United Kingdom, Europe, Australia, and others have returned from Afghanistan and the conflict in Iraq. Between 18 and 30 percent of those returning from war zones to civilian life can be expected to suffer mental health issues, which can lead to family breakdown, homelessness, and other problems. In the United States, for example, 103,792 cases of post-traumatic stress (PTS) have been diagnosed in returned service personnel. M. Audrey Burnam and colleagues have estimated that one in every five military personnel who have returned from Iraq and Afghanistan will develop some form of PTS.[2]

Mental health issues in the defence forces often exist within a culture of stigmatization, with many service personnel reluctant to admit having a problem. Military personnel may not seek treatment for psychological illnesses because they fear it will harm their careers. Even among those who do seek help for PTS or major depression, only about half receive treatment that researchers consider minimally adequate for their illness.[3] Brewin argues that military service can lead to profound changes in identity, affecting both military personnel's perception of themselves and their relationship to the world.[4] These perceptions of the world include disillusionment about human nature in general and a more specific rejection of civilian life. Brewin shows that some veterans report estrangement, with the dominant theme being a sense of being "out in the cold" after leaving the forces and returning to civilian life.[5] Emotional fragility and a loss of confidence and self-worth are prevalent.[6] The transition process is compounded by a loss of purpose and sense of duty, service, and belonging to a tight-knit team.

This chapter is informed by my work on The Difficult Return: Arts-Based Approaches to Mental Health Literacy and Building Resilience with Recently Returned Military Personnel and Their Families, a four-year interdisciplinary research initiative (2012–14). The project, funded by an Australian Research Council Discovery grant, is a sister project to the Contact!Unload initiative. As part of the research, we developed practice in three areas: 1) awareness – online digital films using a range of strategies, including music; 2) motivation – the development of The Return, a research-based theatre piece featuring ex-servicemen and actors;[7] and 3) action – the Veterans Transition Program (VTP), a psycho-educational program that used elements of role play and enactment, developed in partnership with the University of British Columbia (UBC), Canada.[8] There has been continued close collaboration with UBC researchers: initially, Marv Westwood and his team came to Australia to run two VTP programs and deliver training, and then, following the production of our play, we provided advice to George Belliveau on the early development of Contact!Unload.

Our experiences of implementing these projects with veteran support organizations and ex-service personnel and their families, and our close collaboration with the University of British Columbia, led me to consider international practice and the extensive history of how the arts and military have been used in different ways over time. In this chapter, I provide some context for current policy and practice in the area of arts and health with veterans, and also trace some of the antecedents of how arts-based approaches have been integrated into the history of a developing understanding of combat-related stress (in all its definitions) and its treatments.

Policy and the Recent Growth in Arts Practice

One of the most critical policy initiatives in arts, health, and the military sector in the last few years has been the establishment of the National Initiative for Arts and Health in the Military in the United States. This initiative has hosted four summits (the most recent in 2017) and published a white paper, a national policy action plan, a database, and a toolkit for artists working with veterans.[9]

The transition needs of military personnel has also been explored in the United Kingdom with the continuing work of Combat Stress and a new research hub as part of the Veterans and Families Institute for Military Social Research, Anglia Ruskin University, Cambridge. So while the term "sector" should be used tentatively, the social imperative to explore ways of supporting transition and resilience in the military is the focus of substantive international interdisciplinary work.

Much of the recent arts practice with veterans has developed from a complementary and/or third-sector space (e.g., outside of or marginal to "official" programs). Often these spaces are surprising to both the artist and the veteran community. For example, it would be difficult to mandate the Royal Danish Ballet dancers to work with veterans, or the development of choral music with veterans in an addiction setting.[10] In our own work developing a documentary theatre performance with ex-servicemen and actors, it has been surprising to see how adept soldiers are at performing and how readily audiences from a military background respond to and engage in the arts. These insights are repeated and deepened here in this book, collecting the impressions, ideas, and reflections of how the arts were "deployed" in *Contact!Unload*, a project that built on Marv Westwood's pioneering group work in applied counselling and the use of action-based approaches to re-enactment.

The associated growth in arts and health practice has aligned strongly with the development of grassroots, veteran-led community organizations. These organizations have often developed out of veterans' sense of frustration and a desire for advocacy and better supports and services. Veterans' organizations typically range from small to medium-sized and work on a not-for-profit basis, operating in a range of ways. In the United States, there are organizations like Dry Hootch, which operates a drop-in centre, group counselling, and a "dry" place to hang out with other veterans. Similarly, in Australia, there are organizations such as Young Diggers and Stand Tall, which have an online information and advocacy site as well as a drop-in centre that includes clinics about dealing with Veterans Affairs claims and benefits, activities, social nights, and camps. A more formal initiative has been Mates for Mates, funded as a one-stop shop for veterans and their families and offering a gym, outdoor pursuits, counselling, and other forms of support. The existence of such organizations is significant because as soon as personnel move out of the military, there are often numerous issues with seeking administrative or financial support and aftercare. While departments such as Veterans Affairs (in the United States) and Veterans' Affairs (in Australia) exist to provide benefits, they are often viewed by veterans as overly bureaucratic organizations.[11]

Contemporary arts and health practices often grow out of these associations with veteran groups who are looking for a wide range of opportunities and options for their members, rather than from formal sections of the military. However, forums such as the National Initiative for Arts and Health in the Military and projects like *Contact!Unload*, demonstrate that senior military personnel are increasingly open-minded about and interested in the potential of new approaches.

An important perspective that is missing from the general debate is non-Western approaches to working with returning veterans. There has been significant work in this area, particularly with returning child soldiers in Africa and some work in Colombia.[12] I suspect there is considerably more work in non-Western contexts, and an important next step would be to document and assess how different cultures explore this territory.

In a sense, the link between the arts and the military has been intimately tied to the impact of combat on individuals. The political and social history of psychological and medical terms for combat-related mental health injuries is an important one to understand, as the arts, as previously mentioned, have been used both as an intervention and as a response by soldiers to deal with trauma.

The extraordinary achievements documented in this book highlight some of the ways in which artists, psychologists, counsellors, and military veterans can collaborate together to deal with the kinds of issues that post-deployment produces. One of the surprising elements of arts/military practice and its history is the ways in which a collaborative approach to "treatment" has been foregrounded. The braiding together of different kinds of knowledge – psychiatry, psychology, counselling, the lived experience, and aesthetic modes of doing (theatre, dance, music) – is what makes the contemporary practice and its history such a rich area of endeavour.

The Emergence of a Condition and Early Arts Interventions

The intersections between theatre and the military date back to the very beginnings of theatre history. The Greek tragedies were all written in a sixty-year time span during which Athens was consistently at war.[13] The plays were often written by citizen-soldiers for mass audiences of citizen-soldiers and generals, and often focused on war and its traumatic aftermath. Rather fascinatingly, the theatre of Dionysus was situated adjoining the healing sanctuary of Asclepius so that the songs of the chorus and healing potential of the plays could be heard by the recovering soldiers.[14] The impact of war has been richly represented in poetry, plays, and music from these early days of antiquity. However, while arts-based forms of healing and treatment have been evidenced in subjugated forms of knowledges, it was not until the First World War that they entered into formal medical diagnosis.

Previously called war neurosis, shell shock, battle fatigue, soldier's heart and nostalgia, and other names, post-traumatic stress disorder (PTSD) was formally acknowledged in 1980 and recently rephrased as post-traumatic stress (PTS); this recognition grew out of pressure from professionals and from American Vietnam veterans who were suffering from the disorder.[15] Since 1980, the term has become a unifying concept for a wide range of traumatic experiences, such as child abuse, rape, natural disasters, torture, and war. The main symptoms of PTS include:

- re-experiencing symptoms, such as flashbacks, intrusive memories, and dissociative experiences
- avoidance symptoms, including numbing, isolation, and avoidance of reminders of the traumatic event
- hyper-arousal symptoms, including sleep disturbance, anxiety, anger, impulsivity, and increased startle responses.[16]

These symptoms were documented and identified for the first time in any comprehensive way during the First World War. "Shell shock" emerged as an acknowledged term, although initially it was thought to be the result of a physical injury to the nerves and exposure to heavy bombardment. The war poet Siegfried Sassoon (1983) describes the psychological experience of shell shock in his poem "Survivors." He writes of soldiers with "dreams that drip with murder" and their "stammering, disconnected talk."[17]

Shell shock was often perceived as a sign of emotional weakness, and soldiers were routinely convicted of desertion from duty and, in certain cases, shot by their own side for cowardice. French physicians were the first to conclude that shell shock was essentially a psychological phenomenon.[18] British military physicians divided the classification into two categories: shell-shocked wounded (those exposed to direct physical trauma) and shell-shocked sick (those for whom there was no exposure to direct physical trauma).[19] The First World War undoubtedly produced a major shift in recognizing and evaluating "combat stresses." A report written in 1915 by Company Quartermaster Sergeant Gordon Fisher reflects the change in attitude:

I went further along and looked into the next dug-out and there was a guardsman in there. They talk about the psychology of fear. He was a perfect example. I can see that Guardsman now! His face was yellow, he was shaking all over, and I said to him, "What the hell are you doing here?" He said, "I can't go. I can't do it. I daren't go!" Now, I was pretty ruthless in those days and I said to him, "Look, I'm going up the line and when I come back if you're still here I'll bloody well shoot you!" ... when I came back, thank God, he'd gone. He was a Coldstream. A big chap six-foot tall. He'd got genuine shell shock. We didn't realize that at the time. We used to think it was cowardice, but we learned later on that there was such a thing as shell shock. Poor chap, he couldn't help it. It could happen to anybody.[20]

Despite the growing recognition of shell shock as a psychological condition, the treatment of it was diverse and often severe, including solitary confinement, electric shock treatment, shaming, physical re-education, and emotional deprivation. Treatment of enlisted men tended to be harsher than that of officers.[21] The context of these treatment ideas and therapies was a political need to develop quick and effective approaches in order to return as many men as possible to combat.[22] However, many of these radical treatment methods were not used with officers in the British Army. Typically, officers were encouraged to rest and were withdrawn from the battlefield for longer periods. Nascent forms of psychoanalytical approaches were experimented with and were accompanied by appeals to repress fears and encourage patriotism and loyalty. This highlights some of the contradictory treatment modalities of psychiatrists at the time, and the ways in which the hierarchical nature of the military infused the working medical approaches to managing shell shock.

Many county lunatic asylums, private mental institutions, and disused spas were taken over and designated as hospitals for mental diseases and war neurosis. By 1918, there were more than twenty such hospitals in the United Kingdom. One of the most progressive hospitals was Seale Hayne in Devon, under the directorship of Dr. Arthur Hurst. Hurst developed a range of therapeutic approaches with a focus on positive and purposeful activities. Patients were taken to the countryside for walks and undertook voluntary work on local farms. Hurst promoted creative projects such as listening to music, painting, and writing and producing a ward magazine. He also experimented with re-exposure to guns by taking patients shooting and initiated combat reconstructions to help the men relive their experiences under controlled conditions. One of these exercises was caught on an extraordinary piece of film, called *Re-enacting the Battle of Seale Hayne,* which was directed, photographed, and acted by convalescent war neurosis patients.[23] The rationale for Hurst's work foreshadows the development of occupational therapy in focusing the patient on purposeful rehabilitation. It also pre-empts psychotherapeutic approaches to PTS treatment, which include hypnosis as well as implosive therapy and flooding techniques that try to desensitize the client to the trauma while in a relaxed state.[24]

The political imperative for treatment during the First World War was to get the military personnel fit again for further engagement. The widespread acceptance (evidenced by the establishment of specialist hospitals) of shell shock as a medical condition during the war appeared to wane during the immediate postwar period, driven perhaps by cost and pensionability issues. Many of the medical officers who testified during the British War Office Committee on Shell Shock in 1922 perceived the phenomenon as cowardice or of manipulation to obtain discharge from the danger zone.[25] In the postwar United States, the condition was described as "pension neurosis," and was even attributed to certain ethnic groups.[26] There was considerable hope that the lessons learned about shell shock and its treatment in the First World War would usher in a new period of modern approaches to mental health. Unfortunately, at an institutional level, the lessons of war took time to manifest amid the economy drives and evaporation of postwar idealism.[27] Despite this, there were a number of indices of hope that emerged directly from the treatment of shell shock. The Mental Treatment Act of 1930 was a progressive development at the time, as was the founding of two new institutions, the Cassel Hospital in Merseyside and the Tavistock Clinic in London, dedicated to treating mental health in the general population but informed by wartime practices.

The interwar years are often considered a period of regression and forgetfulness in terms of lessons learned about war neurosis. There was an active attempt to separate, and indeed dismiss, cases of neurosis that arose after the war. Francis Prideaux, a psychiatric expert for the Ministry of Pensions, reported that any claim for "delayed shell-shock made after seven years was clearly bogus."[28] Ben Shephard argues that Prideaux's report, on the eve of the Second World War, was clearly designed to "lock medical policy machine into a very restrictive definition of war neurosis."[29] The Second World War did re-engage military and psychiatric treatments, but with perhaps more emphasis on the use of drugs and hypnosis. There are some small examples of arts-based approaches during this period, but they are more diffuse than the early experiments during the First World War.

The reluctance of governments and the military to accept the validity of war neurosis under any definition has continued. An acceptance of the condition, of the effects and impact of conflict, has considerable implications at a political, military, and societal level. The fight to acknowledge PTSD (as it was then known) in the late 1970s was born out of a culture of official negation, bureaucratic backsliding, and concern about the economic and legal implications of defining such a condition.

Responding to Vietnam: The Development of Treatment Programs for US Veterans

The nature of combat-related PTS clients differs from that of patients suffering from non-combat-related PTS.[30] While PTS sufferers in general are often victims of an event, military personnel may be both perpetrators and victims. This may lead to a moral injury: "the lasting psychological, biological, spiritual, behavioral, and social impact of perpetrating, failing to prevent, or bearing witness to acts that transgress deeply held moral beliefs and expectations."[31] Many combat veterans develop PTS as a result of traumas they have caused, such as killing people. Veterans are also likely to have experienced sustained exposure to traumatic experience over weeks and months. Further, the ontological impact of engaging in legitimized acts of violence, authorized and sanctioned by the nation, places an individual in a complex and confusing moral and immoral, legitimate and illegitimate weave. This can present profound challenges for medical interventions because the symptoms are not just emotional or cognitive, but deeply moral and philosophical in that a patient may be suffering from the commission of unspeakable atrocities.[32]

In the case of Vietnam veterans, the conditions are complicated by the length of the time it took to get support and treatment. These veterans often suffer from what is referred to as the "secondary trauma of return."[33] This form of PTS is only indirectly related to the original trauma and is connected to the hostile reception of troops returning from Vietnam after the war, leading to maladaptive patterns that often led to internalized blame.

Much of the more developed arts practice grew out of the Vietnam War, where formal recognition and definition of terms such as "PTS" led to more sustained interventions and programs. M. James and D.R. Johnson developed drama-based programs with Vietnam veterans in a Veterans Affairs medical centre in the United States.[34] The drama element was integrated with other creative therapies, including visual arts, music, and poetry.[35] The program consisted of three phases: 1) process (e.g., safety through dramatic play); 2) practice (e.g., rehearsal of coping behaviours using role play); and 3) autobiographical performance for an invited audience (reconnection with the world).

Johnson's approach is underpinned by developmental transformations through which patients are encouraged to develop trust in an improvisational playspace.[36] The major focus of developmental transformations is not the specific reliving or problem solving of life experiences, nor achieving catharsis, but rather embracing an attitude of acceptance and tolerance of the multifaceted aspects of the self, good and bad, profound and superficial. The goal becomes to expand the freedom that the individual has in moving from one level of experience to another, rather than the ability to work out one particular conflict.[37]

The chronic nature of PTS has also led to different phases of treatment over time. D.R. Johnson, S.C. Feldman, S.M. Southwick, and D.S. Charney identified the need for the development of First and Second Generation programs in which initial treatment focuses on core PTS symptoms, while follow-up work emphasizes the reintegration of veterans into the social context of family and employment.[38] They state:

> First Generation programs aim to provide a corrective emotional experience for Vietnam veterans, by being highly responsive to their needs, recognizing their entitlement to services previously not given, and by welcoming them back home with respect. These programs emphasize a review of the war, particularly the primary traumas, and management of the core PTSD symptoms of re-experiencing, avoidance, and hyper-arousal.[39] The optimal environment for First Generation work occurs when the treatment setting is experienced as a sanctuary in which their special needs are attended to, and they are given a great deal of support. The primary task of the therapist is listening to their story. Hope is generated by the idea that if you can "get it out," your load will be lightened, and your recovery can begin.[40]

Second Generation programs lead on from these processes, but focus on the present and future rather than the past. Heterogeneous groups rather than homogeneous groups are formed in which veterans are encouraged to make connections outside of the Vietnam trauma circle:

> Traumatized persons need to abandon their identity of being a victim. This requires active re-exposure and attention to other people's lives, interests, and difficulties ... It is crucial to avoid the formation of a group of victims united against a dangerous world, with an idealized leader who will protect the members against further harm.[41]

The concept of First and Second Generation interventions helps to map out a discourse of the ways in which the chronic needs of people with PTS shift over time. Within a medical paradigm, arts-based therapies have quickly established themselves as contributing to an integrated approach to the needs of people with combat-related PTS.[42] As with the work of Hurst and the early pioneers, the arts have been used not just as recreation but in exploring the ways in which "traumatic memories are coded nonverbally in kinaesthetic and visual forms."[43]

Johnson observes that play is often conspicuously absent in PTS patients.[44] The job of the therapist is to maintain the playful environment (defined as a space in which emotions can be played out). Therefore, the therapist moves from "leader-directed to group determined structures, from simple to complex activities, from actions of low to high interpersonal demand and from relatively impersonal to more affectively-laden content."[45] Similar drama therapy programs with combat-related PTS patients have been documented, in particular, Marty Mulkey's work with male veteran survivors of sexual assault.[46]

Besides the drama-based therapeutic group processes that have been explored by a number of practitioners, there are other forms of performance that have been utilized in the combat-related PTS field. J.P. Wilson, A. Walker, and B. Webster have explored the use of ceremony, drawing heavily on Native American rituals of purification for returning warriors.[47] There are obviously difficulties in transferring these types of ceremonies to other cultures, particularly since part of their efficacy is drawn from the cultural ownership and traditions of the veterans' background. However, these uses of ceremony indicate the significance of ritualized behaviour in signalling and representing a transition in expectations for veterans and the community. In Western cultures, rituals of procession and welcome-home parades have been used consistently to acknowledge returning and remembered veterans.

The work of Johnson and colleagues also encompasses ceremonies that focus on the loss of veterans' friends in the war.[48] The researchers created a ceremony with a veteran treatment group that took place at the Vietnam memorial on Long Island Sound. Each veteran brought a piece of paper and a poem, a prose work, or items of remembrance. The ceremony honoured veterans' friends and included the burning of paper to symbolize their ashes. Incorporating the memorial in the ceremony highlights the ways in which these sites of remembrance are used, especially by Vietnam veterans, to seize a link with the past. While the work of Johnson and colleagues is part of an integrated approach within a therapeutic context, it is intriguing to note the ways in which memorials, as aesthetic symbols, exist as sites for informal rituals of mourning and loss. The Vietnam Veterans Memorial in Washington, DC, is a minimalist V-shaped panel with roughly 58,000 names inscribed in 140 plates. It is one of many such memorials, but it is the only site in Washington where artifacts are left.

Visitors to the memorial scrutinize the panels looking for names familiar to them, unable to refrain from touching what they read, and they leave behind (at the base of the walls or wedged into a seam) flowers, letters, women's under-pants, teddy bears, model cars, photographs, and even a Harley-Davidson motorcycle. Maya Lin, the designer of the wall, believed that the names them-selves would be the Vietnam veterans' memorial, requiring no embellishment. What she did not take into account was that mourners would try to give to these names the keepsakes of identity, as if to restore to the dead the intimate worlds they had lost.[49]

> These keepsakes number more than 40,000 and initially were labelled "Lost and Found," until the park authorities realized that they were being left intentionally. These objects, most of them left anonymously, are now taken to a warehouse, catalogued, and stored. In so doing the Park Service has transformed them "from individual artifacts to aesthetic objects of memory."[50]

While memorials are officially sanctioned spaces of mourning and remem-brance, the informal response to the Vietnam Veterans Memorial wall is para-doxically intimate and communal. Like the containing form of the ceremony, the wall seems to offer a structured (physical and spiritual) space for mourners and the dead. It offers a (sanctioned) space in which to communicate and com-mune with the dead. The informal response, never an intention in the construc-tion or the design of the wall, signifies an important area in which the arts often exist outside of medical paradigms. Both have their value. The work of Johnson and colleagues is an example of a highly imaginative treatment intervention that draws on different aesthetic modalities.[51] The wall offers an insight into subjugated ways of knowing in dealing with the chronic nature of combat-related stresses and the PTS condition.

An alternative history of arts with returned military personnel is provided by the examples of the private impulses to make art as a response to combat and PTS. These are not the sanctioned work of war artists or compelling re-sponses by artists viewing the war from afar, but rather the poetry, songs, art, and theatre that emerged from the trench, or the difficult return home from combat zone to civilian life.

Contemporary Arts, Health, and Military Practice

As evidenced by the chapters in this collection, there is a growing interest and diversity in the field of arts and health in military contexts. Arts and health practices are either integrated within mainstream treatment modalities or exist as alternatives to more traditional psychiatric and psychological (e.g., cognitive behaviour) approaches.

Many claims have been made about the impact of arts and culture in the context of military-related trauma, but there is also considerable skepticism about the evidence base of the arts. It is not clear precisely which components of a therapy are necessary and which components lead to treatment success. The creative therapies often utilize multimodal designs where patients engage in both creative and cognitive components, making it difficult to establish what specifically caused the positive effects. As the number of treatment sessions ranges from three (expressive writing) to upward of a hundred (art and multimodal therapies) and follow-up intervals vary, it is not clear how much of each treatment is necessary for symptom reduction or how long the effects of a given treatment may last.[52]

The evidence from the project described in this book illustrates the importance to participants of working through the arts to build and strengthen protective health factors. The circumstances of deployment typically provide the raw material for participants' engagement in the various creative activities as outlined in the following chapters, but they also offer an opportunity for veterans and their families to understand and negotiate the difficulties involved in the process of transition back to civil society. *Contact!Unload* clearly works at multiple levels in supporting participants to articulate and deal with feelings of isolation and to develop their self-sufficiency and resilience. It also advocates for therapeutic models that are appropriate, and that protect confidentiality, for returning veterans who have suffered psychological stress injuries during combat. The theatre piece is able to show the group-based therapeutic model, enabling audiences to witness not only the injuries but ways of healing for veterans when given proper care.

In evaluating the Difficult Return project in Australia and comparing it with the achievements in *Contact!Unload*, it's possible to identify the central qualities where the arts and military experience might interconnect.[53] One of the potential benefits of these projects is the centrality of story and meaning making in understanding the self and our place in the world. In working with *homo narrans* – the storytelling primate – it is possible to see how language and representational action have given us a significant survival advantage as a species.[54] From the Greeks onward, there has been an instinct to use theatre and performance as a form of catharsis and integration of difficult stories. The modes and forms have changed and developed, but the fundamental principle persists. Through processes of integration like the Veterans Transition Program, there can be insight and, importantly, emotional catharsis through the release of a story that had become trapped in the body. Importantly, the VTP provides not only a release but also a defined process of integration and regulation of the participants' psychosocial functioning. This step in the process is critical, and neither the Difficult Return project nor *Contact!Unload* would have been practicable without it. The performance of unresolved stories in a public forum by ex-servicemen, given the right ethical contexts, can add a further dimension to the work. Our experience with the performance project within the Difficult Return research was that it enabled an aesthetic transformation that led to a higher level of integration and a collective resonance between performers and audience. In performing a story onstage, the ex-servicemen felt that they were able to transform their story into something else, where the focus was on empowerment, creativity, and spontaneity.

Perhaps one of the most compelling outcomes of the performance was that other veterans dealing with mental health issues saw the men onstage as role models for what might be achievable. The staging of their stories thus became, for some of the soldier-actors, an act of moral revival in which the trauma story and the journey towards change shifted how they saw themselves from moral victim to role model. The performance enabled them to review how their own personal story might be contextualized in a public forum, and reinforced a strength-based view that storytelling could be experienced as a way of reintegration with the broader community.

Notes

Material in the chapter was previously published in Michael Balfour and Donald Stewart, "Perspectives and Contexts of Arts, Social Health and the Military," *Arts and Health* 7, 2 (2015): 87–95, https://doi.org/10.1080/17533015.2014.999247.

1 T. Nadelson, "Journey of Healing: An Outpatient Therapy Group for War-Related PTSD," *Psychiatric Services* 50, 5 (1999): 627.

2 M. Audrey Burnam, Lisa S. Meredith, Terri Tanielian, and Lisa H. Jaycox, "Mental-Health Care for Iraq and Afghanistan War Veterans," *Health Affairs* 28, 3 (2009): 771–82.

3 T. Tanielian and L.H. Jaycox, eds., *Invisible Wounds of War: Psychological and Cognitive Injuries, Their Consequences, and Services to Assist Recovery* (Santa Monica, CA: RAND, 2008).

4 C.R. Brewin, "The Nature and Significance of Memory Disturbance in Posttraumatic Stress Disorder," *Annual Review of Clinical Psychology* 7 (2011): 203–27.

5 Ibid.

6 Ibid.

7 L. Hassall and M. Balfour, "Transitioning Home: Research-Based Theatre with Returning Servicemen and Their Families," in *Research-Based Theatre: An Artistic Methodology,* ed. George Belliveau and G.W. Lea, 103–16 (Bristol: Intellect, 2016).

8 M. Balfour, M. Westwood, and M.J. Buchanan, "Protecting into Emotion: Therapeutic Enactments with Military Veterans Transitioning Back into Civilian Life," *Research in Drama Education: The Journal of Applied Theatre and Performance* 19, 2 (2014): 165–81, https://doi.org/10.1080/13569783.2014.911806.

9 National Arts Administration and Policy Publications Database (NAAPPD), http://www.americansforthearts.org/by-program/reports-and-data/legislation-policy/naappd/arts-deployed-an-action-guide-for-community-arts-military-programming.

10 J. Bowman, "'Wounded Warriors': Royal Danish Ballet Dancers Train Repatriated Wounded Soldiers in Pilates," *Arts and Health* 7, 2 (2015): 161–71; M. Liebowitz, M.S. Tucker, M. Frontz, and S. Mulholland, "Participatory Choral Music as a Means of Engagement in a Veterans' Mental Health and Addiction Treatment Setting," *Arts and Health* 7, 2 (2015): 137–50.

11 K.W. Kizer and A.K. Jha, "Restoring Trust in VA Health Care," *New England Journal of Medicine* 371, 4 (2014): 295–97.

12 T.S. Betancourt, S. Simmons, I. Borisova, et al., "High Hopes, Grim Reality: Reintegration and the Education of Former Child Soldiers in Sierra Leone," *Comparative Education Review* 52, 4 (2008): 565–87; J. van Kesteren, "Acting for Peace: Participatory Theater in Peace Education in Colombia" (master's thesis, University of Amsterdam, 2011).

13 T.G. Palaima, "When War Is Performed, What Do Soldiers and Veterans Want to Hear and See and Why?" in *Combat Trauma and the Ancient Greeks*, ed. P. Meineck and D. Konstan (New York: Palgrave Macmillan, 2014), 261–85.

14 B. Doerries, *The Theatre of War: What Ancient Greek Tragedies Can Teach Us Today* (London: Scribe, 2004).

15 J. Miller and D.R. Johnson, "Drama Therapy in the Treatment of Combat-Related Post-Traumatic Stress Disorder," *The Arts in Psychotherapy* 23, 5 (1997): 383–95.

16 B. van der Kolk, *Psychological Trauma* (Washington, DC: American Psychiatric Press, 1987).

17 S. Sassoon, *The War Poems* (London: Faber and Faber, 1983), 35.

18 D.H. Marlowe, *Psychological and Psychosocial Consequences of Combat and Deployment with Special Emphasis on the Gulf War* (Santa Monica, CA: RAND, 2000), http://www.gulflink.osd.mil/library/randrep/marlowe_paper/index.html.

19 A. Babington, *Shell Shock: A History of the Changing Attitudes to War Neurosis* (London: Leo Cooper, 1997).

20 Cited in L. MacDonald, *1915: The Death of Innocence* (New York: Henry Holt, 1995), 476.

21 J. Ellis, *Eye Deep in Hell: Trench Warfare in World War I* (Baltimore: Johns Hopkins University Press, 1984).

22 Marlowe, *Psychological and Psychosocial Consequences of Combat*.

23 *War Neuroses: Netley 1917, Seale Hayne Military Hospital 1918* (United Kingdom: Pathé, 1918). At least three versions of the film exist. There are copies at the Welcome Trust Moving Image and Sound Collection, the BFI National Archive, the Imperial War Museum, and British Pathé (currently managed by ITN).

24 H. Crasilneck and J. Hall, *Clinical Hypnosis: Principles and Applications* (Orlando, FL: Grune and Stratton, 1985); J.A. Lyons and T.M. Keane, "Implosive Therapy for the Treatment of Combat-Related PTS," *Journal of Traumatic Stress* 2, 2 (1989): 137–52.

25 E.J. Leed, *No Man's Land: Combat and Identity in World War I* (Cambridge: Cambridge University Press, 1981).

26 G.H. Benton, "'War' Neuroses and Allied Conditions in Ex-service Men," *Journal of the American Medical Association* 77, 5 (1921): 362.

27 B. Shephard, *A War of Nerves: Soldiers and Psychiatrists 1914–1994* (London: Jonathan Cape, 2002), 161.

28 Ibid., 166.

29 Ibid.

30 M. James and D.R. Johnson, "Drama Therapy in the Treatment of Affective Expression in Posttraumatic Stress Disorder," in *Knowing Feeling: Affect, Script, and Psychotherapy*, ed. D.L. Nathanson, 303–26 (New York: Norton, 1996).

31 B.T. Litz, N. Stein, E. Delaney, L. Lebowitz, et al., "Moral Injury and Moral Repair in War Veterans: A Preliminary Model and Intervention Strategy," *Clinical Psychology Review* 29 (2009): 697, https://doi.org/10.1016/j.cpr.2009.07.003.

32 S.A. Haley, "When Patients Report Atrocities: Specific Treatment Considerations of the Vietnam Veteran," *Archive of General Psychiatry* 30, 2 (1974): 191–96.

33 James and Johnson, "Drama Therapy," 385.

34 James and Johnson, "Drama Therapy."

35 R.L. Blake and S.R. Bishop, "The Bonny Method of Guided Imagery and Music (GIM) in the Treatment of Post-Traumatic Stress Disorder (PTSD) with Adults in a Psychiatric Setting," *Music Therapy Perspectives* 12, 2 (1994): 125–29; C. Dintino and D.R. Johnson, "Playing with the Perpetrator: Gender Dynamics in Developmental Drama Therapy," in *Drama Therapy: Theory and Practice*, ed. S. Jennings, 3: 205–20 (London: Routledge, 1996); S. Feldman, D. Johnson, and M. Ollayos, "The Use of Writing in the Treatment of PTSD," in *The Handbook of Post-Traumatic Therapy*, ed. M.B. Williams and J. Sommer, 366–85 (Westport, CT: Greenwood, 1994); James and Johnson, "Drama Therapy."

36 D.R. Johnson, "The Role of the Creative Arts Therapies in the Diagnosis and Treatment of Psychological Trauma," *The Arts in Psychotherapy* 14, 1 (1987): 7–13; Dintino and Johnson, "Playing with the Perpetrator"; James and Johnson, "Drama Therapy."

37 James and Johnson, "Drama Therapy," 385.

38 D.R. Johnson, S.C. Feldman, S.M. Southwick, and D.S. Charney, "The Concept of the Second-Generation Program in the Treatment of Post-Traumatic Stress Disorder among Vietnam Veterans," *Journal of Traumatic Stress* 7, 2 (1994): 217–35.

39 F. Gusman, *Description of Specialized PTSD Program at VA Medical Center* (Menlo Park, CA: n.p., 1990); R.M. Scurfield, "Post-Trauma Stress Assessment and Treatment: Overview and Formulations," in *Trauma and Its Wake*, vol. 1, *The Study and Treatment of Post-Traumatic Stress Disorder*, ed. C. Figley, 219–55 (New York: Brunner/Mazel, 1985); S. Silver, "An Inpatient Program for PTSD: Context as Treatment," in *Trauma and Its Wake*, vol. 2, *Traumatic Stress Theory, Research, and Intervention*, ed. C. Figley, 213–31 (New York: Brunner/Mazel, 1986).

40 Johnson et al., "The Concept of the Second-Generation Program," 226.

41 van der Kolk, *Psychological Trauma*, 165.

42 D. Golub, "Symbolic Expression in Post-Traumatic Stress Disorder: Vietnam Combat Veterans in Art Therapy," *The Arts in Psychotherapy* 12, 4 (1985): 285–96; Johnson, "The Role of the Creative Arts Therapies"; C. Malchiodi, *Breaking the Silence: Art Therapy with Children from Violent Homes* (New York: Brunner/Mazel, 1990); S.L. Simonds, *Bridging the Silence: Nonverbal Modalities in the Treatment of Adult Survivors of Childhood Sexual Abuse* (New York: Norton, 1994); M. Bensimon, D. Amir, and Y. Wolf, "Drumming through Trauma: Music Therapy with Post-Traumatic Soldiers," *The Arts in Psychotherapy* 35, 1 (2008): 34–48.

43 James and Johnson, "Drama Therapy," 384.

44 Johnson, "The Role of the Creative Arts Therapies."

45 James and Johnson, "Drama Therapy," 385.

46 M. Mulkey, "Recreating Masculinity: Drama Therapy with Male Survivors of Sexual Assault," *The Arts in Psychotherapy* 31, 1 (2004): 19–28.

47 J.P. Wilson, A. Walker, and B. Webster, "Reconnecting: Stress Recovery in the Wilderness," in *Trauma, Transformation, and Healing: An Integrated Approach to Theory, Research, and Post-Traumatic Therapy,* ed. J.P. Wilson, 159–95 (New York: Brunner/Mazel, 1989).

48 Johnson et al., "The Concept of the Second-Generation Program."

49 P.S. Hawkins, "Naming Names: The Art of Memory and the NAMES Project AIDS Quilt," *Critical Inquiry* 19, 4 (1993): 755.

50 M.B. Junge, "Mourning, Memory and Life Itself: The AIDS Quilt and the Vietnam Veterans' Memorial Wall," *The Arts in Psychotherapy* 26, 3 (1999): 199.

51 Johnson et al., "The Concept of the Second-Generation Program."

52 J. Smyth and J. Nobel, *Arts and Healing: Creative, Artistic, and Expressive Therapies for PTSD* (White Paper) (Brookline, MA: Foundation for Art and Healing, 2011), 3, http://www.artandhealing.org/wp-content/uploads/2015/07/PTSD-White_Paper_0323121.pdf.

53 Hassall and Balfour, "Transitioning Home."

54 M. Warner, *Stranger Magic: Charmed States and the Arabian Nights* (London: Vintage, 2012).

2

Contact!Unload
The Cauldron

Chuck MacKinnon

CONTACT!UNLOAD: a short title that encapsulates so much more.

Two words, two meanings. Two worlds collide, meld, and become the colloquial brass ring for many others ...

Where was I before this all started ... Who was this veteran before the performance?

Anxiety, hesitation, pain revisited. Not only your own but others'. Through the use of the dialogue from the play and imagery, try in a brief chapter to let the audience understand the journey. Apparently, the dialogue cannot solely be based on the word *Fuck*. However, comedian George Carlin may disagree ...

The dialogue was so personal, a woven fabric of time and experiences. It shaped the production crew, the performers and veterans, and the audience, both civilian and veteran.

Encapsulate your experience, they ask ... but where to start? I was a veteran thankful for the previous counselling that I had experienced, well, sort of. The counselling sessions became a lantern in a torrid storm of pain, emotion, and confusion. Once by land; twice by sea ... Paul, you make it sound easy. Be careful, the light at the end of the tunnel or journey could be a train ...

Why would anyone keep hammering their hand with a hammer? Do it once, they say, is bad, repeating the same thing with the same results – crazy. So, why did we do it? Why did we keep opening our wounds in front of audiences? Like *Contact!Unload*, three principles guided veterans: Mission first, Men second, Self last. Your Mission, if you choose to accept it, is to help others. One of our ways of helping was to share our stories with audiences, including other veterans.

A pebble in a pond, touching others, reaching out, touching the anguished souls of veterans, the victims or bystanders of death by suicide, giving understanding, nay, insight. Having those who watch feel your pain if only for a moment. Our thespian journey transcended the edges of our stage for we are merely actors within it.

3

Facilitating Therapeutic Change through Theatre Performance

Alistair G. Gordon, Marv Westwood, and Carson A. Kivari

> *Your battles inspired me – not the obvious material battles but those that were fought and won behind your forehead.*
>
> – JAMES JOYCE

DESCRIPTIONS OF THE TURMOIL that can follow soldiers home from war are nothing new. From Herodotus's character Epizelus at the Battle of Marathon (Greek), Lucretius's poem *De Rerum Natura* (Roman), the *Gisli Sursson Saga* (Icelandic), to Jean Froissart's chronicling of the Hundred Years' War, military trauma has informed stories for millennia.[1] While the experience of psychological injury may remain constant, our language to describe it certainly does not. Last century alone, the "irritable heart" of the American Civil War became the First World War's "shell shock," reflecting the neurological damage often caused by heavy artillery.[2] The Second World War transformed our language again to "combat stress reaction" and "combat fatigue." The psychiatric community has, for now, settled on "post-traumatic stress" – a term we can at least for now agree on.

Regardless of the changes in description, the blindness that Epizelus suffered despite "neither having received a blow in any part of his body," John Rambo's grief-induced hypervigilant flashbacks in the movie *Rambo: First Blood,* and the guilt that plagues the soldiers in *Contact!Unload* are enduring and consistent experiences of war.[3] They are the archetypal sufferings of the warrior that outlast mere description.

It is fortunate, then, that treatment for combat-related traumatic stress has evolved just as much as the terms used. In the First World War era, common interventions included electroshock therapy, hydrotherapy, and hypnosis. During the Second World War, a common treatment was PIE (proximity, immediacy, and expectancy), a practice more concerned with keeping soldiers in battle than with their healing from it.[4] Since then, the trend towards evidence-based therapies, including exposure, cognitive processing, and eye movement desensitization and reprocessing (EMDR), has helped shape the field.[5]

Of great interest to us, however, are group-based interpersonal approaches and dramatic enactments – perhaps less mainstream interventions that nonetheless can powerfully integrate traumatic injury.[6] Emerging most prominently following the Vietnam War, action-based dramatic therapies have since undergone a period of rigorous intentional structuring to enhance their psychotherapeutic value.[7]

The use of theatrical enactment in soldiers' healing should come as no surprise, as military personnel and civilians have long engaged in drama within conflict zones by witnessing performances of plays.[8] This tradition has evolved in the present with military-themed productions such as *Fallujah,* an opera depicting Sergeant Christian Ellis's struggles with post-traumatic stress.[9] Similarly, plays in this genre are often charitable and research-oriented, such as *Shell Shock.*[10] This play is adapted from the 2011 book by the same name, depicting fictional Corporal Tommy Atkins's failing career and relationships in the context of postwar trauma.

The *Contact!Unload* project further advanced this idea by casting veterans themselves (i.e., non-actors) as performers. This was an intentional therapeutic intervention, guided by psychologists and clinical counsellors. When real soldiers are used, the safety of clinical supervision is unequivocally necessary. It is Virgil's hand, guiding Dante through the rings of hell that he may find his Beatrice.[11] This is no metaphor, because in telling their stories, the activation of traumatic stress symptoms may constitute an all-too-real "return to hell." Our veterans make this sacrifice so that there may be greater peace for themselves and others.

The Great Return

The soldiers who performed in *Contact!Unload* experienced trauma to a degree that many civilians can never fully grasp. Performing their stories risks activating terrible and overwhelming feelings. Traumatic stress is stored in the body, as it were, often resulting in feelings of helpless dread during high stress (such as performing publicly).[12] Certainly, we could see this in our performers. Shaking hands and voices, nausea and dizziness. "Fight or flight" systems "hijacked" their conscious experience at a moment's notice, suggesting through their feelings that they should run for their lives. What is more remarkable is that they didn't.

Such a dramatic return to the time and place of their wounding, performed for mostly civilian strangers no less, required a clear motivation. The veterans reported that their primary motivation was to build awareness among their peers about the challenges and hopes of returning to civilian life. They also reported wanting to inform and educate the public about the lived experience of veterans (see Chapter 2), a world mostly hidden from others. In other words, they sacrificed comfort in the moment so that others could better understand with increased patience and compassion. This is an act of service for returning soldiers who may feel monstrous or may lack the words to explain to their family their wild behaviours. Focus groups suggested that this increase in understanding extended not only to veterans but also to individuals in general who were experiencing mental health struggles.[13]

Veterans also reported participating to extend their own healing – that is, they continued the therapeutic benefit from their initial participation in the Veterans Transition Program (VTP), the therapeutic intervention on which *Contact!Unload* is based.[14] Like Hercules in the throat of the sea monster or Pinocchio in the belly of the whale, our veterans tolerated the hardship of re-visiting their traumas for the treasure that was to come (i.e., transformation of self and audience), facilitated by the theatrical development process and performances.

The Alchemy of Suffering

A major part of the play's therapeutic benefit is catharsis. Catharsis may be defined as a sudden shift of perception (i.e., insight) and a surge of emotion(s) (e.g., grief, anger, or sadness) connected to previously hidden memories from "old psychological wounds."[15] The result is the understanding and grieving of traumatic losses in a manner resonant not only with the audience but also reportedly with the performers.[16]

The theatrical space culminates in a cacophony of emotive output as collective anguish emerges in a dance of chaos becoming order. Put poetically, unseen amorphous pain takes shape as visible scar tissue, moving from the shadows of the past to the bright splendour of the present, evaporating under rays of understanding and newly made meaning. Put in clinical terms, implicit memories are grieved publicly as painful unconscious memories emerge into conscious awareness, mitigated by public compassion that allows positive insights and change to emerge.

A significant aspect of catharsis as we have described it in the context of performance may be "embodied simulation," a neural process by way of mirror neurons.[17] The "monkey see, monkey do" adage describes how mirror neurons often prompt our intentions, actions, and even emotions to parallel those of others through visual cuing.[18] This process could help explain why the feeling states of theatre performers and audience members frequently mirror each other in a synchronized emotive community. In this case, the therapeutic value of theatre is manifested as a mirroring of performers and audience members that informs a subtle (and not so subtle) cathartic experience.[19]

The personal control, safety, and group cohesion that emerged during the development of *Contact!Unload* enabled the veterans to experience their emotionally laden memories and beliefs in new ways. Previously hidden and often painful memories emerged into conscious awareness and were paired with new realizations. While this process is now supported by modern neuroscience, it also echoes the great psychoanalytic traditions of Sigmund Freud and Carl Jung, on which modern psychotherapies were built: *Make the unconscious conscious.*[20]

This emergence of experience into conscious awareness is the opposite of what occurs during real-time trauma. During moments of profound terror, experience is imprinted implicitly (i.e., unconsciously) in the form of memories that largely operate on somatic, sensory, and procedural levels – that is, they are subtle and automatic, emotionally reactive, and beyond language. This is what B.A. van der Kolk means by *The Body Keeps the Score* – the title of his influential book on how trauma directly impacts the body systems.[21] With theatre, these hidden body memories emerge into conscious awareness within the social container of public compassion and empathy from fellow actors and audience members. This leads to the potential for positive change.

Beyond Trauma Repair

Other mechanisms of theatre performance also create positive change for performers. For instance, part of what creates the safety required for catharsis as described above is the climate of acceptance that supports performers to act out what may be considered morally wrong. In the rehearsal and performance spaces, a community bears witnesses to the veterans' beliefs, thoughts, emotions, actions, and memories. The performers may then receive understanding, normalization, acceptance, and, perhaps most importantly, social connection. Because the need to be seen, heard, and understood that is fundamental for psychological health is met, the veterans are then able to process their experience while reconciling moral injuries.[22]

The language that we choose also helps to facilitate healing. An important component of military trauma repair is using words that soldiers themselves would use (e.g., "fuck"), especially since clinical and academic word choices may be stigmatizing and repelling.[23] This emerged naturally in the early days of the VTP, as the complex process of trauma repair was affectionately labelled as "dropping the baggage."

Dropping the baggage is not the only healing process that takes place in theatre. The practice of behavioural rehearsal, for instance, is a staple of recovery in therapeutic enactment, the drama-rooted core intervention of VTP.[24] Repeating an action with important personal meaning (e.g., practising assertiveness or vulnerability) can heighten personal competence. This increases self-efficacy, the belief that one can achieve one's goals and create desired change.[25]

Self-efficacy not only raises behavioural competence but can also lower social fear by increasing individuals' likelihood to approach social situations they previously avoided due to unrealistic and catastrophized fears (e.g., "There is something deeply wrong with me that everybody can see"). These anxieties are lowered because the reality of the present in the rehearsal disproves old beliefs, which often resulted from earlier life experiences (e.g., severe bullying creates the mistaken belief that adults will continue the vicious behaviours of children).

The Closest Thing to Real

Theatre performance can provide the lived experience of situations that helps to reduce traumatic stress, challenge unrealistic and negative beliefs, and support a positive self-image.[26] The proximity and similarity of performance to real-life events may be key to change, contrasting therapeutic approaches that rely strictly on changing conscious thought processes (e.g., cognitive reprocessing).[27] Trauma is not talked or thought into the body, but enacted through potent and overwhelming events.[28] Therefore, the activation of as many psychological processes as possible (e.g., cognitive, emotional, verbal, perceptual, and sensorimotor) through enacting a context similar to the original with adaptations including regulation, developing constructive behaviour, and meaning making is thought to underlie the mechanism of change. The theatre is a space where new endings can be written, both metaphorically and literally.

The rehearsals and performances of *Contact!Unload*, as described in this book, offer a form of therapeutic lived experience characterized by present-focused, interpersonal action that can lead to a myriad of effects on both the individual and the group. This results in the integration of the following domains: 1) physiological – decreased anxiety; 2) relational – positive and meaningful interactions and multiple responses from other performers and audience members; 3) cognitive changes – greater perceived confidence in self; and 4) emotional expression – a subjective sense of calmness and satisfaction from increased self-confidence and reduced anxiety.

Performance also has the advantage of constructing and representing traumatic events in ways that may not be possible in classical therapeutic settings.

On top of this, conventional therapy almost never takes place with an audience (usually for good reason!). Performing with witnesses, however, may produce a microcosm of society, leading to greater conviction of perceptions attained during dynamic simulated lived experiences and interpersonal interactions. It is the absolution from the public court that is often overwhelmingly relieving for those whose guilt feels unforgivable.

The Final Act (Revised)

The traumatic wounding of warriors has been represented across the ages through literature. The experience of postwar suffering that we currently call post-traumatic stress has remained consistent, unlike our language to describe it and the approaches to helping those experiencing it. The performance and rehearsal of theatre are powerful catalysts for the healing and education of performers and patrons alike.

While the visible effects are self-evident, an academic lens reveals multiple benefits of theatre. Catharsis and empathy are vehicles for the conscious emergence of buried and implicit imprints of painful events. Feeling seen, heard, and understood repairs connection to community, while rehearsal of bold and adaptive actions undoes fearful avoidance. Of great importance, theatrical performance closely parallels the dynamic social, emotional, and behavioural experiences involved in real-life events – an enduring vehicle for Dr. Marv Westwood's legacy of therapeutic enactment and the core of the therapeutic initiative used by the Veterans Transition Network (http://www.vtncanada.org).

While this chapter began by paralleling our work to classical literary accounts of soldiers, there is one striking feature that distinguishes *Contact!Unload* from historical texts. That is its focus on hope and healing. Thank you to all involved in the project who have helped rewrite history, providing *the possibility of a happy ending!*

Notes

1 M.-A. Crocq and L. Crocq, "From Shell Shock and War Neurosis to Posttraumatic Stress Disorder: A History of Psychotraumatology," *Dialogues in Clinical Neuroscience* 2, 1 (2000): 47–55.

2 E. Jones and S. Wessely, *Shell Shock to PTSD: Military Psychiatry from 1900 to the Gulf War* (New York: Psychology Press, 2005).

3 Epizelus: R.D. Morritt, *Echoes from the Greek Bronze Age: An Anthology of Greek Thought in the Classical Age* (Newcastle upon Tyne: Cambridge Scholars Publishing, 2010), 53. John Rambo: B. Feitshans (producer) and T. Kotcheff (director), *Rambo: First Blood* (Anabasis N.V., 1982), motion picture, 93 minutes.

4 E. Jones and S. Wessely, "'Forward Psychiatry' in the Military: Its Origins and Effectiveness," *Journal of Traumatic Stress* 16, 4 (2003): 411–19, https://doi.org/10.1023/A:1024426321072.

5   C.L. Lancaster, J.B. Teeters, D.F. Gros, and S.E. Back, "Posttraumatic Stress Disorder: Overview of Evidence-Based Assessment and Treatment," *Journal of Clinical Medicine* 5, 11 (2016): 105, https://doi.org/10.3390/jcm5110105.

6   For example, M. Balfour, M. Westwood, and M.J. Buchanan, "Protecting into Emotion: Therapeutic Enactments with Military Veterans Transitioning Back into Civilian Life," *Research in Drama Education: The Journal of Applied Theatre and Performance* 19, 2 (2014): 165–81, https://doi.org/10.1080/13569783.2014.911806; D.W. Cox, M.J. Buchanan, S.M. Hoover, and M.J. Westwood, "Re-experiencing Military Trauma in Groups: A Veteran's Case Study," *Canadian Journal of Counselling and Psychotherapy/Revue canadienne de counseling et de psychothérapie* 48, 4 (2014): 441–53; M.J. Westwood, H. McLean, D. Cave, W. Borgen, and P. Slakov, "Coming Home: A Group-Based Approach for Assisting Military Veterans in Transition," *Journal for Specialists in Group Work* 35, 1 (2010): 44–68, https://doi.org/10.1080/01933920903466059.

7   M. Balfour, "The Difficult Return: Contexts and Developments in Drama-Based Work with Returned Military Personnel," *Applied Theatre Researcher/IDEA Journal* 10 (2009), http://hdl.handle.net/10072/30005. For a more detailed discussion, see the Introduction.

8   J. Thompson, J. Hughes, and M. Balfour, *Performance in Place of War* (Calcutta: Seagull Books, 2009).

9   "Fallujah: The Opera," YouTube video, posted by Explore Documentary Films, May 27, 2016, http://www.youtube.com/watch?v=HPZ9SHjb40A.

10 T. Marriott, *Shell Shock* (Sussex, UK: Shell Shock Media, 2017).

11 Alighieri, Dante, *Divine Comedy* (1320; repr., Richmond, UK: Alma Books, 2018).

12 B.A. van der Kolk, "The Body Keeps the Score: Memory and the Evolving Psychobiology of Posttraumatic Stress," *Harvard Review of Psychiatry* 1, 5 (1994): 253–65.

13 G. Belliveau and J. Nichols, "Audience Responses to *Contact!Unload*: A Canadian Research-Based Play about Returning Military Veterans," *Cogent Arts and Humanities* 4, 1 (2017), https://doi.org/10.1080/23311983.2017.1351704.

14 D.W. Cox, M.J. Westwood, S.M. Hoover, E.K.H. Chan, et al., "The Evaluation of a Group Intervention for Veterans Who Experienced Military-Related Trauma," *International Journal of Group Psychotherapy* 64, 3 (2014): 367–80.

15 US Department of Health and Human Services, Substance Abuse and Mental Health Services Administration, *Brief Interventions and Brief Therapies for Substance Abuse* (Rockville, MD: Department of Health and Human Services, 2012), 168, https://www.ncbi.nlm.nih.gov/books/NBK64947/pdf/Bookshelf_NBK64947.pdf.

16 B.W. McLean, "*Contact!Unload*: A Narrative Study and Filmic Exploration of Veterans Performing Stories of War and Transition" (master's thesis, University of British Columbia, 2017), https://doi.org/10.14288/1.0343358.

17 A. Cook, "Interplay: The Method and Potential of a Cognitive Scientific Approach to Theatre," *Theatre Journal* 59, 4 (2007): 590, https://www.jstor.org/stable/25070112.

18 V. Gallese, M.N. Eagle, and P. Migone, "Intentional Attunement: Mirror Neurons and the Neural Underpinnings of Interpersonal Relations," *Journal of the American Psychoanalytic Association* 55, 1 (2007): 131–75, https://doi.org/10.1177/00030651070550010601; M. Iacoboni, "The Human Mirror Neuron System and Its Role in Imitation and Empathy," in *The Primate Mind: Built to Connect with Other Minds*, ed. F.B.M. Waal and P.F. Ferrari, 32–47 (Cambridge, MA: Harvard University Press, 2012).

19 It should be noted that this process also took place during rehearsals and was not limited to performance.

20 On support from modern neuroscience, see, for example, L. Cozolino, *The Neuroscience of Human Relationships: Attachment and the Developing Social Brain* (New York: W.W. Norton, 2014). Freud and Jung: S. Freud, "Zur Dynamik Der Übertragung" [The dynamics of transference], *SKSN* 4 (1918): 388–98; C.G. Jung, "On the Psychology of the Unconscious," trans. R.F.C. Hull, in *The Collected Works of C.G. Jung*, vol. 7, *Two Essays on Analytical Psychology*, 2nd ed., ed. G. Alder and R.F.C. Hull, 1–119 (Princeton, NJ: Princeton University Press, 1968; originally published 1917).

21 B.A. van der Kolk, *The Body Keeps the Score: Brain, Mind, and Body in the Healing of Trauma* (New York: Viking, 2014).

22 R.F. Baumeister and M.R. Leary, "The Need to Belong: Desire for Interpersonal Attachments as a Fundamental Human Motivation," *Psychological Bulletin* 117, 3 (1995): 497–529, https://doi.org/10.1037/0033-2909.117.3.497; D. Umberson and J.K. Montez, "Social Relationships and Health: A Flashpoint for Health Policy," *Journal of Health and Social Behavior* 51, 1 (supp.) (2010): S54–S66, https://doi.org/10.1177/0022146510383501.

23 C.A. Kivari, J.L. Oliffe, W.A. Borgen, and M.J. Westwood, "No Man Left Behind: Effectively Engaging Male Military Veterans in Counseling," *American Journal of Men's Health* 12, 2 (2018): 241–51.

24 M.J. Westwood and P. Wilensky, *Therapeutic Enactment: Restoring Vitality through Trauma Repair in Groups* (Vancouver: Group Action Press, 2005).

25 A. Bandura, *Self-Efficacy: The Exercise of Control* (New York: Macmillan, 1997).

26 Balfour, "The Difficult Return."

27 Westwood et al., "Coming Home."

28 van der Kolk, *The Body Keeps the Score.*

4
A Soldier's Tale
"Nobody Understood What I'd Done"
Britney Dennison

AMONG THE INVISIBLE *wounds vets carry is guilt born of deadly chaos.*

All soldiers must die in order to live. It's the way the military functions. Fear is a distraction and distractions lead to death. So, as retired signals operator Tim Garthside explains, "You just have to accept that you're already dead. It seems harsh, but if you're worrying about dying, then you're going to die."[1]

The problem is, once you have lived as if you are already dead, it's hard to change back. And it is hard to relate to anyone who hasn't crossed that grimly pragmatic divide.

Tim recalls a ride in an SUV headed for Kandahar Airfield. He and fellow soldiers were escorting non-enlisted support staff who were headed back home. Tim saw the panicked look on the face of one. "He looked like a ghost," Tim says. "I remember laughing in my head like, 'What the fuck is your problem? Why are you so fucking scared?'"

Tim shakes his head. "Then I just sort of started thinking about it a bit later. It's like, 'Why am I *not* scared? What the fuck? Maybe I *should* be scared.'"

Months later, when he returned home, Tim realized that nobody who was there to greet him at the Toronto airport "fucking understood anything about where I'd been. What I'd done."

He isolated himself from everyone he cared about. He moved to British Columbia and gradually stopped speaking to his parents, siblings, and friends. "I spent the majority of my time alone," Tim says. "I didn't experience anything except for my own suffering. And I spent a lot of time contemplating why I was still alive. What the point of me being here was. With no real answers."

"This Cage on Your Head"
Tim was part of the first full Canadian tour in Kandahar, southern Afghanistan. Kandahar is a volatile region.[2] It is the place where the Taliban movement

originated. In 2006, when Tim deployed at the age of twenty-one, the area was seeing a resurgence in Taliban activity.

Tim's job description included operating and maintaining communications systems. His location was a small camp in the middle of Kandahar with the Provincial Reconstruction Team. Some days he patrolled with the military police, and he liked that. "I didn't want to be stuck in the headquarters." In fact, it was at headquarters where "the real traumatic things that really crushed me happened," Tim says. "All my trauma came from sitting in an office chair with headphones on." He was the guy in charge of hearing all the signals going back and forth and letting everyone know what was going on. The headphones were Tim's prison. "It's like you're wearing this trap," he says. "This cage on your head all the time."

Tim was the voice troops relied on if they were in harm's way outside the wire. On August 3, 2006, four Canadian soldiers were killed and ten wounded when one bomb blew up a convoy and a second exploded amid the first responders. After the explosions the troops began receiving enemy fire from a nearby compound. Tim was on the line, receiving communications from the battle. There was nothing he could do. He couldn't help the injured and dying while they were in the middle of a firefight.

"When you call for a medevac, part of the deal is, 'Are they taking fire?' And if they're taking fire then the helicopter is not coming," Tim says. "So, I was the one telling them repeatedly that no one's coming. They just kept asking."

Tim has written about that day. In an article published by the BC/Yukon Command Legion, he wrote: "As their life source poured from their bodies and they slowly and painfully breathed their last breaths, I was the one denying them any hope of survival."

For years Tim agonized from having to repeatedly say, "No one is coming." But while he was there, while he was in it, there was no room for emotions. "When you listen to a radio transmission there's never any emotion," Tim says. "Where does it go? It goes into the guy saying it."

In trying to save his men, Tim spoke with air support, poised to come in and help clear out the enemy. There was no time to waste because once the enemy was gone Tim could then send the medical evacuation so desperately needed. Two attack helicopters were sent up. They were relying on counter-intelligence for information on where and who to target. Counter-intelligence had a source on the ground who could confirm the location of the compound, so through that source Tim was able to tell the pilots where to go and who to kill.

At one point, one of pilots saw a man standing on a roof with a rocket-propelled grenade. He asked Tim, "Should we kill him?" Tim's answer was yes – if the man had an RPG (rocket-propelled grenade), then yes, they should.

So, they did. "They cut him in half. Their words, not mine," Tim says.

Then counter-intelligence notified Tim they'd lost contact with their source on the ground – the phone was dead.

It turns out the man on the roof was their source. "I ordered that guy to be killed who was helping us," Tim says. "Who was essentially saving those lives that were standing there needing help. I killed that guy."

At the end of his shift, his boss asked if he was okay. His reply: "Of course I am."

"That Tipping Point"

I'm fine. I'm okay. Those words are like a soldier's mantra. Tim came home barely three weeks after the terrible day of August 3, 2006. His recurring self-statement was always, "I'm fine." He kept telling himself that since he'd never been shot at or hit by an improvised explosive device (IED), he couldn't be traumatized.

But he was.

He quit the military eight months after returning from Kandahar and ended up in Coquitlam, BC, where he found work as a crane mechanic. His work became his life. He would get up. Go to work. Come home. Not talk to anyone. Sit alone. Go to bed. Wake up and do it all again. "I wasn't Tim," he says. "I was the job."

But once Tim was past the steep learning curve that becoming a crane mechanic demands, he was left with more time to ruminate. "It progressively just got worse over the years," Tim says. "I just turned into this tumultuous ball of emotion. And I was getting really angry all the time and I'm just not an angry person."

Tim had never heard of a trigger before. He thought his panic attacks were because he smoked too much. He thought he was out of breath because the equipment was heavy. The triggers kept getting worse – he was jumpy, on edge – he wasn't himself. Then came a day – in September 2012.

"I was just extremely unstable. I could barely keep myself from crying. I just seemed sort of on that tipping point all the time between anger and grief and I was just in pain." On his coffee break, Tim phoned Veterans Affairs. "I just asked for help. I was like, 'Look I've served. I'm a veteran. I served in Afghanistan in 2006. I don't know what to do anymore. I'm at the end of my rope. Nothing

I'm doing is working. I'm thinking about killing myself. I don't know what to do. I need help. I don't need help tomorrow. I need help now.'"

The voice on the other end of the line told him to "print out a form and mail it to us then we can help you."

Tim left work, but he didn't own a printer. So he went to the Legion and had them print off the form for him. The man printing the form told Tim there was an Afghan veteran there and asked if he'd like to talk to him.

That's how Tim met his friend Aaron, who's a graduate of the Veterans Transition Program (VTP) at the University of British Columbia. "I didn't have to talk to him about it really. He could just see where I was at," Tim says. Three weeks later he was in the program.

"If it hadn't been for that I probably would have killed myself." Tim stares out the window for a moment. "I would not be here."

"They Saw Things"

Tim has been diagnosed with post-traumatic stress disorder (PTSD) and major depressive disorder. Sitting in his apartment, Tim leans over and pets his dog Monty. He looks lost in his memories, lost in his story. It's a story that lives and breathes within him, and one that he's told countless times.

The first time was to Marv Westwood, a counselling psychologist at the University of British Columbia and a co-founder of the VTP.

"I'll never forget my interview with Marv," Tim says. "I seriously smoked an entire pack of cigarettes before I went in."

Tim still wasn't sure he belonged. He wasn't sure how he could be traumatized. He felt fearful of opening up. But Westwood "just asked me where I'd served and what I'd done," Tim says. "There was something about him that put me at ease. I felt like I was being understood, and that hadn't happened for me for a really long time."

Westwood says there are wounds not caused by explosions or gunshots. "Some in the military service will let you know that they saw things and did things they shouldn't have. And the innocence is lost," he says. "The soul injury, the loss of self, they are invisible and yet they are very dominant."

No soldier or veteran is fine, Westwood says. "That's denial. It's part of their military masculine culture. There's a lot of people who do need help and some of them kill themselves or stay depressed and isolated."

But it doesn't have to be that way. Recovery and restoration is possible. Westwood told Tim he was like an iceberg – he'd been frozen for a long time and he was just now beginning to thaw.

Lock and Key

The VTP is designed for soldiers to help soldiers. "Nobody comes back without wounds. If you go you've been hurt," Tim now sees.[3] "So, the basis of that brotherhood is that you've been through hell. And you come out the other side, and you probably have scars – you do." It was the validation of those scars by fellow soldiers that helped Tim acknowledge his trauma and begin to work through it.

The program is offered over three months. Its focus is on storytelling and re-enacting those stories to reach a resolution. Westwood says they start by focusing on the positives – by talking about what they gained and what they learned while overseas.

Then they focus on losses. They call it "dropping baggage."

Each person identifies a story or a loss they had during their military experience. They tell the story. They write it out and then they re-enact it.

Tim says his therapeutic enactment forced him to go back to the August 3 disaster and switch back on something that had been turned off that day. "That was really the first time that I'd felt emotion in seven years," Tim says. "A lot of it just involved getting angry and then once I got that anger out of the way there was just grief. A lot of grief."

The metaphor Tim was given was that if you stick your hand in a snowbank it freezes. When you take your hand out, the first thing you feel is burning and pain. That's what going back feels like. "Before you can feel any of the good stuff you're going to feel all of the bad stuff," he says. "You are back feeling those same things, and then you can slow it down and deal with the emotions. You do whatever you need to do to release that stuff."

Tim's second enactment was about acknowledging all the pieces of himself he'd lost in Afghanistan. It was about confronting the Tim he was before. The Tim that was drawn to the army before he learned the army would ask him to die in order to stay alive.

During this enactment there was an empty chair across from him. Tim put his soldier self in that chair. And he didn't hold back. "You fucking lied to me," he said. "You told me about the honour and the valour and the truth and all this horse shit, and you didn't tell me about what I'm going to have to fucking carry around for seven years. You didn't tell me any of that stuff. You fucking lied to me."

Tim has done several enactments since starting with the VTP in the fall of 2013. His third enactment brought him back once again to August 3. This time Tim realized he blamed himself for what happened to the man on the roof. All of his self-criticism came rushing back. It was like someone was standing behind him telling him, "You're a monster. You're terrible and you deserve this."

Tim's counsellors asked, "What would you say if it was somebody else standing there? Do you feel bad for him?"

Tim answered, "I'd tell him that it's not his fault, but it is. It is his fault. I'd want him to feel better but ..."

Then they asked, "So this person just has to suffer forever because of this?"

Westwood can't offer Tim any kind of memory-erasing cure. "You have to remember what you did forever and what you saw," he says to Tim. "But you don't have to suffer from that forever."

Hearing that, Tim says, "just gave me the hope that I can be forgiven even if I can't forgive myself. You can almost hear a lock being turned."

"Who I Am Now"

What motivates soldiers to share their story? Marv Westwood believes they want to give back. If they think telling their story can help someone else, they will. And it will help them heal their own wounds. "What they can get back after they drop the baggage, is that they can actually begin to feel hopeful. They begin to imagine that they can have careers. They can have a family. So, they can get those things back – their goals and their aspirations."

With Canada's combat mission in Afghanistan at its close, veterans will increasingly need help transitioning to civilian life. In 2012, the number of suicides in the US military surpassed the number of soldiers killed in combat – suicides rose to 349, nearly one a day, while combat deaths in Afghanistan numbered 310. In Canada, a study released in 2013 says there were 10 military suicides in 2012. But these numbers are deceptive. Only suicides by male regular force personnel are officially recorded – the statistics don't include suicides by women, veterans who are retired, or reservists.

Tim was in the reserves, so if he had killed himself, as he says he often contemplated doing, he would not have been counted among those official statistics.

Now Tim is back in school. He's completing an undergraduate degree in social work at the University of Victoria. He also supports the Veterans Transition Network, which has expanded to six provinces across Canada and has more than 900 graduates in nine provinces. The program, he says, "saved my life."

Tim has been doing everything he can to turn his suffering into something positive. But he expects the trauma will never go away.

"PTSD is a blanket that goes over my brain and it affects everything. It's just reality for me," he says.

In the face of his suffering there is one question Tim gets asked more than others: "Would you do it again?"

His answer is always "yes."

When Tim deployed he believed in the mission. He believed that by going he could make a difference. He says he felt ready to do something, change something, and be part of something much bigger than himself.

Tim still feels that way. "Things get twisted and turned around and politicized and whatever else, and at the end of the day nothing's perfect," he says. "But we did help people, for whatever small amount of change that may have fostered."

What these soldiers are finding is that there is pain that destroys and pain that transforms. Tim says his scars are a reminder of what it means to be alive. "If I had to go back I wouldn't change a single thing about it because it's made me who I am now," he says.

"Regret gets you nowhere."

Notes

This story originally appeared on November 10, 2014, in *The Tyee* as part of a three-part series profiling three veterans seeking, in their own ways, healing from war's invisible wounds (https://thetyee.ca/News/2014/11/10/Soldiers-Tales-Told/). It has been lightly edited for inclusion in this volume, and all endnotes are editorial contributions added by the editors of this volume. Graham Lea, lead scriptwriter, was greatly influenced by this article when writing *Contact!Unload*.

1 See Moment 5 in the Annotated Playscript in this volume.
2 Some of Tim's quotes in this section were adapted into Moment 21.
3 Some of Tim's quotes in this section were adapted into Moment 21.

5

Listening through Stories
Insights into Writing *Contact!Unload*

Graham W. Lea

TO REFLECT THE PERSONAL and sometimes messy experiences of co-developing *Contact!Unload,* I share this chapter as a series of journal entries based on the notes and observations I made while writing the play, as well as photos, videos, and memories. These entries are not intended to provide a step-by-step description of the writing process, nor are they exhaustive. Rather, they highlight some key motivations, moments, and tensions, as well as personal, professional, and pragmatic issues and questions I encountered and struggled with during the development process. These entries in conjunction with the script aim to shed light upon some of the thinking that went into the development of *Contact!Unload* from my role as an artist on the project.

Entry 1: Vancouver, Fall 2015 – A First Discussion

I have been asked to co-develop a research-based theatre script highlighting the work of the Veterans Transition Program (VTP). There seems to be a strong interest in mounting a full production, which greatly interests me. I haven't had a chance to fully stage any of my previous research-based theatre scripts. This project has funding, institutional support, and the explicit intent to create a performance. A full production will allow me to more fully explore my desire to use theatre to express research. George Belliveau, a member of the research team, is also interested in how elements of theatre such as dialogue, lighting, sound, and ritual might be used in research.[1] There'll be encouragement for more than just a "talking heads" performance or a script full of monologues.

That said, there are constraints. There is a budget but it isn't that big. Lots of stakeholders to navigate. Only four months to devise and mount the play, working mostly on weekends. I will also be stage-managing the final production. Moving from writer to stage manager is something I haven't done before and may cause some challenges. So how is my involvement in this project to work? What do they want of me? I think they want someone to:

- observe and participate in development sessions
- identify key stories, script them, and find a way to frame them as a thirty-minute play
- avoid cliché
- create something disruptive and engaging.

George suggested looking at Pirandello's *Six Characters in Search of an Author* for inspiration for framing the script.[2] This resonates with me as Pirandello's script has inspired much of my curiosity about how theatre makes reality malleable. George is thinking that instead of characters in search of an author, we could have actors in search of a director. Maybe a group of veterans want to perform *Henry V* and need a director?[3] We could incorporate the iconic St. Crispin's Day speech. Definitely something to explore; however, I don't want to predetermine the outcome too much! But any strong starting point is good as we only have four months to devise and stage the play.

Marv Westwood, co-founder of the VTP and a member of the research team, mentioned some key themes that have been identified in their therapeutic work with returning veterans, including:

- grieving – saying goodbye; letting another go
- giving back what was put on you
- taking back – claiming what was originally yours
- saying you're sorry
- survivors' guilt.[4]

I will have to find a way to incorporate some of these into the play somehow. There are a lot of needs to consider for this production even before we start exploring content!

Entry 2: Late Fall 2015

Just came back from my first group meeting at the University of British Columbia. A group of theatre artists, counselling psychologists, and even one of the veterans who might be involved in the project met to talk about how the project might unfold. The neutral-beige room was far from the excitement of a theatre. The world happens in such rooms where plans are incubated only to be hatched somewhere else, somewhere more exciting, more dangerous, more glamorous, more colourful, more ... alive. In the centre of the room, an empty space surrounded by bodies. Peter Brook says that this is all we need to make theatre.[5] But in this empty space, that is not what we make. In this beige room, we sit and make plans for bringing the colours of theatre to the challenges these veterans face.

In preparation, I watched some video clips from the VTP. The stories shared by the veterans in the videos are very difficult; if the ones we encounter are as challenging, I wonder how I might hold and honour them, especially those of trauma. These experiences are pivotal moments in people's lives. Yet to transform them into theatre I might have to alter them, simplify complexities, find an essence. But I might see a different essence. I might have to make cuts, fill in gaps, change language or even the order of events. How can I do this while doing their stories justice? By adapting their stories, do I risk retraumatizing? If so, how do I avoid further harming the veterans who are already dealing with so much? How do I protect them? How do I protect myself? These are personal stories that I am about to help make public. Does this risk reopening old wounds around which a protective scar has developed? I too have had trauma in my life – nothing comparable to what some of the veterans have been through, but challenging nonetheless. How can I hold their stories in a way that does not harm the story, its teller, or me?!

I am both excited and terrified.

Entry 3: Foster Eastman's Studio, February 2015 –
My First Development Session

Second development session today in Foster Eastman's studio. On a flip chart, a list of ideas from the first development session, which I had to miss. I like that we are thinking of a structure from the get-go, but is it too confining? Will it allow the work to grow organically? Does it put the art ahead of the research? Will it overly shape what I observe? What if what I observe doesn't fit within the frame? I will have to be mindful not to be so bound by this structure that I can't let it go. But I must also be aware that thinking this might be the frame will necessarily, even if unconsciously, shape my observations. Should we have waited to allow the frame to emerge from the research? I am both enabled and trapped. Yet in this project we are all, George, Marv, the other "university" members, and I, enmeshed in the research. So perhaps then the frame is indeed emerging from the research.

We began the session today in a discussion circle, working to build a space in which everyone is comfortable engaging in the difficult work ahead. It is interesting that even in these moments I am beginning to hear lines that may find their way into the script. The authentic language of these men is much richer than I can devise:

- The VTP pretty well saved my life.[6]
- I'm fucked up but not that fucked up.[7]
- Injury is injury.[8]

Warren Geraghty (veteran) spoke about the pride he felt that his son had been accepted into the reserves. But despite that, he is still not able to talk about his military experience, even with his now-enlisted son. Interesting how silence shapes us as much as words and action.

During our discussions, Tim Garthside (veteran) described himself as an iceberg, frozen in time.[9] Powerful metaphor ... he can't move, is stuck. At least on some level, I know the feeling. This may be why I am most interested in this project. I couldn't say it in a group but the chance to push the use of theatrical artistry in research-based theatre isn't what really draws me to this project. No, it is more personal, more challenging, more potentially motivational. I too have been haunted. Nothing like what these men have faced, but challenges that have contributed to my not leading the life I want to lead, to my being frozen. Perhaps from them I can gain some techniques, approaches, insights to help bring myself out of the basements, both literal and metaphoric, that I have been living in for way too long. I know I must be open to all stories, not just the ones that resonate with me. There will of course be some conscious and unconscious pull towards those that have personal resonance, but how can I avoid becoming overly biased?

After our introductions, we began our first forays towards theatre. We played "stomp," in which we passed a rhythmic stomp around the circle. Fascinatingly, even though the theatre practitioners had played the game many times before, it was the veterans, new to the game, who had the best rhythm. Tim likened it to being on drill, anticipating people's movements, following and leading. Interesting that this military training emerged and carried over into this simple game.

After observing my first session, I find myself in a very interesting and challenging position. As we talk and do activities, I am both a participant and an observer. The work requires I be involved but I am simultaneously distanced: thinking, watching, being aware of the final product rather than immersing myself in activities. I am an outsider in an insider process. I can't let myself go as much as I would like; perhaps I am feeling the need to maintain some level of distance. Or perhaps my inability to let go is a protection mechanism so that

I don't have to get too close, don't have to open up, don't have to admit that I struggle too but with so much less than they.

Entry 4: Foster Eastman's Studio, February 2015 – A Familiar Feeling

Another session that began with a lot of talking. I find it simultaneously interesting, helpful, inspiring, and frustrating. I get a chance to see these men, their strength, their vulnerability, the strength in their vulnerability. I see their genuine desire to reach out to other veterans, "the silent majority," the ones who are "still alive but they are dead." That is the hook. That is why they are saying, "I'm in," why these military veterans are willing to do something they describe as "artsy-fartsy" as creating a play. But this discussion does not provide much material for me to adapt into the script. How might we rebalance these sessions to focus more on the theatrical development?

One veteran said that before his therapeutic enactment (TE), he "was at the bottom and ... got a hand out." At the bottom, hermited away, a basement. I too have hermited myself. I have spent many days unable to move, to get off the couch, where the sum total of my day was absently watching a marathon of *Storage Wars*.[10]

Just how much of myself can I put into this piece; how much can I take out? I know the impossibility of impartiality. Do I risk making this too personal at the cost of the veterans? How can I allow the research to emerge when I see myself in it? Maybe that is, in some small way, our research ... finding points of intersectionality.[11] To listen through their stories rather than listening to them – to find moments within the specifics of the "shock and awe" of the stories where universalities of struggle might shine through. Perhaps that is my job ... not just to tell the veterans' stories but find ways to make their particulars have a wider resonance without diminishing the horrific things these men have seen ... no easy ask.

During our discussions, Tim expressed his concern that he didn't want this production to turn into "war porn," objectifying stories of horrific events and trauma for a vicarious release or catharsis of the audience. Similarly, Marv wants this production not to be a dark story but rather to show hope and possibility. An idea was floated today that might help with this: dramatizing a TE. This makes dramatic sense. In a TE, veterans re-enact their original trauma.[12] Staging this allows us to show the traumatic event to the audience while simultaneously showcasing the difficult but hopeful work of this therapeutic approach. But the TE is also therapeutic, so this approach provides a way to show rather than tell both the trauma and the potential for healing.

Today, one of the veterans described reaching out to a colleague who was not doing so well. He said that his colleague "needed me to be there for him." I had a thought, a scary one: who am I in this project? Can I be there for them? What does it mean for me to be there for them? Am I even able to do what needs to be done to give everyone the kind of outcome they are hoping for? A lot is resting on these shoulders!!

Entry 5: February 2015, At Break – Questions!

We have just finished the first half of a development session and there is a challenge ... a lot of talk ... talk, talk, talk. Nine people showed up – counsellors, academics, community members – but Dale was the only veteran. Theatre development is not a drop-in, drop-out activity. It needs commitment, especially from those whose stories are to be central to the performance. Are we wasting our time here? Academics can't do this work!!! Even when we had more veterans, we still talked a lot, seemingly more than we engaged in theatre activities. Is therapy overtaking play development? Is play development overtaking therapy? Is working towards a full production (on a tight timeline) getting in the way of both? Are we doing too many things at once? Is there too much time commitment involved for the veterans? There seems to be a natural gravity towards sitting in the circle and talking. I wonder, are we avoiding something? If so, what? Are we being too overprotective? Treating the veterans with kid gloves? Are we researchers too fearful, protecting ourselves from harsh realities in blankets of words? Too scared to risk hurting the veterans, or perhaps ourselves?

We have an academic knowing. The stories I could create from the themes in the literature cannot come close to the real thing. It is stories, their lived knowing, that will give the script authenticity. With these stories I can create a frame to house them and then get out of their way. But how can I build a dramatic frame without knowing what is going into it! Even the *Six Characters in Search of an Author* frame is not working. It feels forced, too complex. There are only six development and rehearsal sessions left. Are we trying to be too clever, showing ourselves off rather than whatever we get from the veterans (if anything)?

Can I come even close to doing this?!

Entry 6: February 2015, after the Session – A Way In

After a mini-crisis of ability at break, I feel a bit more confident in my role in this project. We still had only one veteran but we at least started getting on our feet and working. While I don't yet have any stories, I do have a better idea of how the script might unfold. After a brief warm-up, George led us through the St. Crispin's Day speech. Dale said that the speech feels like bullshit, it rings hollow. Building on this, George had an actor read it again and encouraged the rest of us to interrupt the speech, to speak back to the bullshit. For example, after the line "If we are mark'd to die, we are enow / To do our country loss; and if to live, the greater share of honour,"[13] Dale interrupted the king, asking, "Are you in search of our glory or just yours?"

The interjections felt quite forced; however, the exercise of talking to the speech might provide the frame that is needed. Building on this, the conceit for the script might be that an actor is struggling with the St. Crispin's Day speech and veterans are brought in to help the actor develop authenticity. The veterans can tell the actor what war is really like, and what it is like to return. Through this, the actor moves away from a romantic "ra-ra-ra" style of acting. As the actor develops their understanding, they become a proxy for the audience. It is the actor whose character develops. This simplifies the complexity of the Pirandello frame. When we do eventually get stories, I can then interject them into the St. Crispin's Day speech when I find a resonance between the stories and the speech.[14]

"We few, we happy few, we band of brothers."[15] Today I realized for the first time that Dale has a literal band of brothers, a bracelet inscribed with the names of those who died while he was deployed. As Dale explained in another interjection, it is not for us or for Henry that soldiers go to battle. The cause is not enough; it is the loyalty to the men and women on the left and right. It is the band of brothers and sisters, a bond that extends beyond the battlefield.[16]

Entry 7: March 2015 – Is This the End?
I met with George and JS Valdez (the assistant director) for lunch to discuss directions of the project and script. The script is developing very slowly and I don't feel it yet; I have a rough frame and a few stories from the veterans but nothing enough to sustain an entire performance. While I could create stories that try to capture some of the themes Marv has identified, I don't feel comfortable doing so. My ability is one factor: I know my strengths lie in crafting rather than creating stories. But more important is the ethical challenge. Yes, I have been in difficult personal situations; yes, I have been in very unsafe places; but I have not been in the situations these men have been in. I haven't seen the things they have seen, done what they've done, lost what they've lost. Were I to invent narratives to demonstrate themes, they would be inspired by what little I know of war from movies, TV, news. They would ring hollow. We've been repeatedly told that there has to be authenticity, otherwise veterans in the

audience will disregard the work and possibly dismiss the TE process. They are the audience the veterans most want to reach – those who might benefit from this therapeutic approach. I can't invent authenticity. It has to come from our veterans and I haven't seen enough yet to make a script. And even if I could, were I to invent narratives, I would be taking the work and struggles of these men to tell my story. I would be using their trauma, not helping them express it to others! No, I can't create stories.

As I aired these concerns, I found myself worrying that perhaps I am not the best person for this project. Perhaps, it would be better if I left. Thinking that this might be why they wanted to meet today, to ask me to leave, I offered to withdraw. George seemed to read my angst. Aware of the tight timeline we are on, he suggested that rather than trying to solicit stories from scratch, we try to seed them. Linda Hassall's play *The Return* is based on a similar project in Australia led by Michael Balfour.[17] We could give our veterans scenes from *The Return* to explore as a starting point for development. And if nothing comes out, perhaps scenes from *The Return* could be added to the frame so that we at least have something for the final performance. With this, I am a bit more comfortable with continuing with the project. I have taken a small step back from a precipice.

Entry 8: March 2015 – Seeding Stories

Today we implemented George's idea of seeding the veterans with scenes from *The Return*. We chose several scenes and assigned small groups to work on them. George encouraged us to write on, manipulate, ignore, speak to, or speak against the script to help bring out personal stories. However, there appeared to be deference to the text – I think some thought it was my script. Most groups defaulted to "acting out" the scenes as written, bound by the written text even when given a chance to move beyond it. How powerful the written word.

But some stories started to emerge. For example, Chuck spoke for ten minutes about one of his men who saw a friend killed and then was called to support the family in Canada.[18] I transcribed the conversation and have started adapting it for performance. I am also finding new staging ideas. While I watched a group work on a quiet scene, in the hallway another group was working on a loud and abrasive firefight scene. Hearing these two scenes in jarring juxtaposition, speaking to each other, gave me the idea of presenting them simultaneously? Or perhaps echoes of the loud scene might return in the more sombre scene. How might the various stories speak to each other within the frame? Perhaps a shadow of a tableau or a character from a previous scene might reappear to add a sense of coherence to the piece and commonality to the narratives.[19]

I am becoming increasingly aware of Tim's narrative. I think the notion of being at the bottom and moving towards his eventual TE might be the backbone to this story. I wonder if this is because of my identification with some of this feeling and my using this project to help get out of my own basements. Despite my personal resonance, Tim's experience does provide a way to show the difficult work getting to a TE. His article in *The Tyee* could be adapted into a staged TE.[20] The main narrative would then be Tim's, his move from isolation towards beginning an integrated life through the help of his band of brothers and a TE.

I now have a frame, or rather five interweaving narrative frames, for the production:

1 The overall conceit is an actor and director working on the St. Crispin's Day speech from *Henry V*. The director brings in some veterans to lend authenticity.
2 At certain points during the speech, veterans are triggered. When this happens, they go into a flashback, re-enacting the traumatic memory.
3 After each of these traumatic memory flashbacks, there is a reach-out to the Tim character to try to help him get the help he needs.
4 At the beginning, the Tim character isolates himself. This continues through the play despite numerous attempts to reach out to him. The reach-outs become increasingly assertive until Dale's character, realizing he needs to help his "brother in arms" gives him a marching order to get help: "This is fucking enough."
5 And finally, Tim's TE.

With this frame and some stories, I can start putting a script together. It has been a long and difficult process just to get here. Things may be finally starting to fit together.

Entry 9: March 2015 – Moving Forward

I have now written the first few drafts of a script and we have started to move from development to rehearsal, the part of the process with which I have the most comfort. Yet this is a strange transition for me as I switch roles from playwright to stage manager. I am still more of a playwright right now, focusing on adapting the script based on what evolves during rehearsals. As we move closer to production, I anticipate becoming more of a traditional stage manager, maintaining rather than adapting the script.

I have been searching for a way to meaningfully integrate Foster's Tribute Pole into the play – to bridge the visual art and theatrical components of the

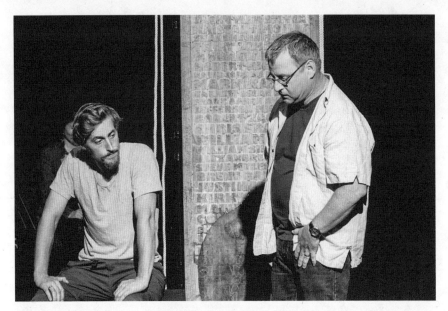

Figure 5 Tim Garthside sitting in front of the Tribute Pole with Chuck MacKinnon during a "Reach Out" moment | Photo by Blair McLean; used with permission.

project. Now that Tim's narrative forms a major part of the play, I think the pole might help tell his story. If Tim is blocked under the Tribute Pole for the bulk of the performance (see Figure 5), then there is a visual reminder of the oppressive weight on those who have returned – a weight not just of those who have died but what returning veterans have experienced while deployed. But Tim's story isn't just one of staying stuck – it is about the hard work to move on a path of reclaiming his life. This journey too can be represented through the staging. If the Tribute Pole is placed upstage right, then Tim spends much of the time in a relatively weak stage position. When he begins the TE, then he moves towards more powerful stage positions centre stage. Then at the end of the performance he exits stage left, as far away from the Tribute Pole as possible. Crossing the stage in this way is powerful as it moves in the same way that we read in English and takes Tim away from being so heavily weighted down, symbolized by the Tribute Pole.

One major challenge I have had developing this script has been Chuck's story about one of his men seeing a colleague killed.[21] How to capture the feeling? How can I understand the difficulty of holding a dying friend? What do you do? What do you say? This week the answer came when I took my cat, Mackie, to the vet for the last time. He has been my closest friend for fifteen years. He travelled across the country with me many times. He was always there for me and trusted me to take care of him. But I couldn't prevent cancer from invading his lungs. I had to say goodbye. After the vet gave the injection, I put my head on his chest and listened. Listened to his breath. In and out, in and out. Getting fainter and fainter until there was no more.

This is my entry point into Chuck's story. Listening to breath. Linda Hassall writes of dramatic fusion, the fusing of the playwright's experiences with other frameworks:

> Fusing the phenomenological with the creative: At the centre of the play is the playwright. ... From the consciousness of the playwright phenomenological discoveries including autobiographical history, lived experience, language and vocabulary and culture emerge. These discoveries are creatively contextualized into dramatic writing which includes symbols, metaphors and images which generate themes, purpose, story and a specific vernacular language.[22]

Few have direct experience with war and combat. It is otherworldly, easy to distance ourselves from the struggles of the men and women who have seen combat. But many of us have experienced loss and challenging periods of transition in our lives. To help bridge this, I fused my experience of listening to my cat's last breaths with that of the soldier in Chuck's story. Perhaps my role in writing this play is not to hold stories, or get out of their way, or shock an audience with the horrors of war. My task is not to listen to stories, it is to listen through them, to find myself in the stories, to reveal universals that resonate in the particular. My role as playwright is to serve as a conduit, a link, between the stories of the field and those of the audience.

Now that the script is taking shape, I too am going through a transition. As I move from playwright to stage manager, my role now is to help bring the script I have created into being as a fully realized performance. As hard as it has been, I am going to miss the writing, miss hearing stories and finding myself within them.

Notes

I would like to thank Dr. Lynn Fels for editorial assistance in preparing this chapter.

1 G.W. Lea and G. Belliveau, "Introduction," in *Research-Based Theatre: An Artistic Methodology*, ed. G. Belliveau and G.W. Lea, 1–12 (Bristol: Intellect, 2016).

2 L. Pirandello, *Six Characters in Search of an Author*, trans. F. May (London: Heinemann, 1954; originally published 1921).

3 B. Mowat, P. Werstine, M. Poston, and R. Niles, eds., *Henry V* (Washington, DC: Folger Shakespeare Library, n.d.), http://www.folgerdigitaltexts.org.

4 M. Westwood, personal communication with the author, June 30, 2016.
5 P. Brook, *The Empty Space* (New York: Touchstone, 1968).
6 See Moment 20 in the Annotated Playscript in this volume.
7 See Moment 11.
8 See Moment 11.
9 See Chapters 4 and 11.
10 See Moment 6.
11 G. Charles, "Worrying about Reconciliation: Building upon Our Commonalities and Our Differences as a Way to Move Forward," in *"Speaking My Truth": The Journey to Reconciliation*, ed. G. Charles, 199–207 (Winnipeg: Aboriginal Healing Foundation, 2018).
12 M.J. Westwood and P. Wilensky, *Therapeutic Enactment: Restoring Vitality through Trauma Repair in Groups* (Vancouver: Group Action Press, 2005).
13 Mowat et al., *Henry V,* IV.iii.23–25.
14 G.W. Lea, "Conditions of Evaluation: Evolving Entry Points for Research-Based Theatre," *Journal of Artistic and Creative Education* 8, 1 (2014): 8–35, https://jace.online/index.php/jace/issue/view/13.
15 Mowat et al., *Henry V,* IV.iii.62.
16 See Moment 19.
17 L. Hassall, *The Return* (unpublished script, 2014).
18 This was adapted into Moment 8. In the original production, it was a monologue. Other voices were added when the production was revisited in the fall of 2015.
19 For an example of this, see the tableau in Moment 8 that returns in Moment 21.
20 B. Dennison, "A Soldier's Tale: 'Nobody Understood What I'd Done," *The Tyee,* November 10, 2014, http://thetyee.ca/News/2014/11/10/Soldiers-Tales-Told/. See Chapter 4 of this volume.
21 See Moment 8.
22 L. Hassall, "Evoking and Excavating Representations of Landscape: How Are Experiences of Landscape Explored in the Creation and Development of a New Play: *Dawn's Faded Rose?*" (PhD dissertation, Griffith University, Brisbane, Australia, 2012), 161, https://research-repository.griffith.edu.au/handle/10072/365436.

6
Suicides to Sydney

Foster Eastman

A RASH OF SUICIDES by Canadian military who served in Afghanistan motivated me to get proactive. I asked myself, "What can I do to help?"

Previous art works I created about Canada's military involvement got the
attention of a few veterans who graduated from the Veterans Transition Network
(VTN). These works included a series of improvised explosive devices (IEDs)
disguised as art pieces. The purpose of this exhibition was to bring awareness
to the fact that IEDs could be manufactured from almost anything; they are
hard to identify and are lethal. The majority of fatalities and injuries inflicted
on soldiers were caused by these homemade devices. I would later hear stories
from veterans about the deadly risks of resting on a wooden bench without first
checking whether an IED was planted in the wall. Bombs could be anywhere
and everywhere. To emphasize this point at the exhibition, I engaged Corporal
Tim Laidler (Ret'd) and Corporal Stephen Clews from the VTN to demonstrate
how easy it is to build an IED.

Another art piece was a Canadian flag created with condiments found in
soldiers' field packs, which also contained their lunch. Every time a Canadian
soldier was killed, I shot the flag with a pellet air gun. Sadly, I shot the art installation 158 times, transforming the Canadian flag into a bloody mess. This piece
was to remind us that Canada was participating in a war where young men and
women were dying or severely injured daily. Because of these works and the
attention they received, I soon met more veterans from the VTN. They introduced me to Dr. Marv Westwood to better understand the mission of the VTN.

This connection with veterans at the VTN and Marv led to the lestweforget-
CANADA mural project, which brought together community members and
veterans to create an art piece recognizing the Canadian soldiers killed in
Afghanistan, as well as to raise funds for the VTN (see Figure 6). The names of
the soldiers were manually transferred onto pages of military training manuals
on canvas panels. Images of women mourning lost lives in Afghanistan painted

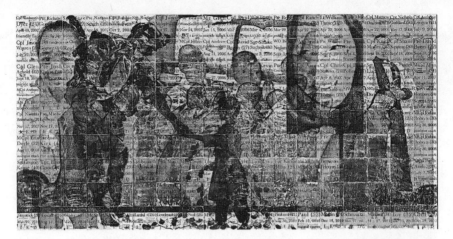

Figure 6 lestweforgetCANADA mural | Photo by Foster Eastman; used with permission.

by a graffiti artist in Kabul were then applied. Images of a ramp ceremony, a mom at her child's funeral, and a child at her parent's funeral were the next layer. The final photo transfer was of a Canadian soldier holding an Afghan boy's hand, symbolizing Canada's entry into and pulling out of the war in Afghanistan.

As they worked together on the art project, conversations between veterans and community members about their experiences developed naturally. Most of the community members involved had never met a soldier before. The environment was safe and intimate, however, allowing for easy conversations about difficult and sensitive topics and experiences. This became a cathartic experience for everyone. I would especially notice when one of the veterans became very quiet while they were working on the panel of one of their friends ... almost as though they were tending their tombstone. Marv soon started to notice that the veterans' mental health had improved, remarking during a hockey game how positive and upbeat the veterans seemed about participating in the art project (perhaps it was the box seats?). Whatever we were doing seemed to be helping. This was a welcome but unintentional by-product of the project. The lestweforgetCANADA mural also raised $120,000 for the VTN.

The mural caught the attention of the True Patriot Love Foundation (TPL), which exhibited it at the National Day of Honour breakfast for families of the fallen in Ottawa, hosted by Prime Minister Stephen Harper in May 2014. It was at this event that family members and military personnel started to sign the backs of the panels with personal notes of love and loss. That November, the mural was showcased in the Canadian War Museum for Remembrance Day ceremonies. It has since been featured at TPL tribute dinners across Canada, with Corporal Stephen Clews and Corporal Dale Hamilton (Ret'd) attending all events and becoming seasoned spokesmen for the project. The mural has also become a significant part of *Contact!Unload*, often touring with the play as a poignant set piece.

This exposure and funding by the Movember Foundation led to the Man/Art/Action project, which aims to reduce men's depression and suicide. One of the components of the project was the use of theatre to help veterans tell their story of transitioning to civilian life, which became *Contact!Unload*. In conjunction with the theatre piece, I worked with master carver Xwalacktun to guide veterans in carving their story into two caskets in what became the Veterans Tribute Pole (see Figure 7).

The Veterans Tribute Pole was aimed at telling stories of soldiers' tours and the challenges they faced once they returned. Military ranks representing the military family were carved into satellite images of Kandahar and Kabul. On the reverse, first names of those killed were carved into maps of Canada. An image of a soldier in distress was then transferred onto the carvings. The caskets were inspired by Indigenous mortuary poles and symbolize the 158 Canadian soldiers who came home in a box and those who feel "trapped in a box" because of depression and operational stress injuries (see Figure 8).

Canadian High Commissioner to the United Kingdom Gordon Campbell asked to exhibit the lestweforgetCANADA mural at Canada House in London. We proposed to showcase the other Man/Art/Action projects as well. With support from the High Commissioner and Brigadier-General Matthew Overton, we were able to highlight both the Tribute Pole and a revised version of

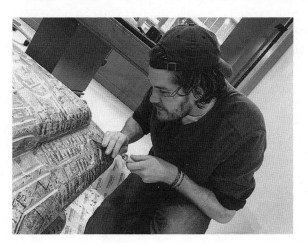

Figure 7 Dale Hamilton carving the Tribute Pole | Photo by Foster Eastman; used with permission.

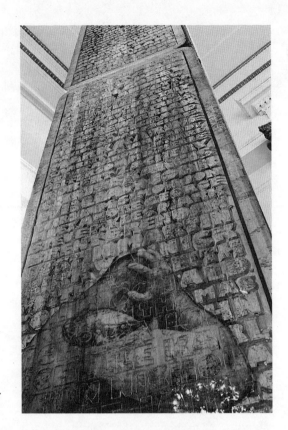

Figure 8 The Tribute Pole in Canada House | Photo by Foster Eastman; used with permission.

Contact!Unload in the fall of 2015. At the time, we didn't realize that a stand-alone mural exhibit is very different from bringing Canadian veterans to perform at Canada House. The logistics required an enormous amount of support from the Canadian military. While in London, these projects attracted royal attention. On November 11, 2015, HRH Prince Harry attended a private performance of *Contact!Unload,* including a ceremonial raising of the Veterans Tribute Pole.

As of this writing, the Tribute Pole stands tall as part of the permanent collection of the Military Museums in Calgary.

In September 2016, the Movember Foundation asked us to share our work at its annual conference in Ottawa. We took this opportunity to also perform *Contact!Unload* at the Royal Military College in Kingston, at Parliament Hill for members of Parliament, and at the Canadian War Museum.

Movember generously provided some funding to help bring our team, including veterans, artists, and academics, to participate as part of the cultural programming of the 2017 Invictus Games in Toronto. With such a large project, however, we needed to search for supplemental sources of funding. One of these sources was the development of the SERIOUSshit art project.

Similar to the lestweforgetCANADA mural, veterans and community members were invited to my studio in order to create an art piece. The idea was to explore how feelings about the war in Afghanistan translated into colour and colour placement. Each participant was issued a waste alleviating gel (WAG) bag and instructed to write their thoughts about Canada's involvement on the toilet paper and deposit those words into the WAG bag. Participants then sorted through reclaimed waste paints and chose colours that best referenced those feelings. Those paint colours were deposited into the WAG bag, and participants placed the bag somewhere meaningful to them on a six-foot canvas with an image of a Canadian soldier in full combat gear. Using an air pellet gun replica of a Canadian military C7A2 automatic rifle, they shot the WAG bag and evacuated the contents onto the canvas. Participants sponsored their canvas in order to take part in this art project. With their generosity and participation, we were able to raise the remaining funds necessary to showcase our work at the Invictus Games. Over eighty canvases were created for the SERIOUSshit installation, which recognizes the Canadian soldiers who died by suicide after returning home from service (see Figure 9).

During the Invictus Games, we showcased the lestweforgetCANADA mural, the SERIOUSshit project, and five performances of *Contact!Unload*. These included performances at the Canadian Institute for Military and Veteran Health Research, the Moss Park Armoury, and the host hotel for the Invictus Games.

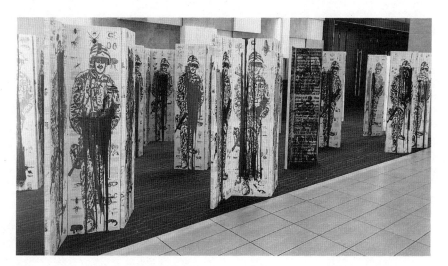

Figure 9 Panels from SERIOUSshit | Photo by Foster Eastman; used with permission.

George Belliveau and Marv were also invited to present this work with veterans at the 9th International Arts and Health Conference at the Art Gallery of New South Wales and at the Big Anxiety Festival at the University of New South Wales in Sydney, Australia. Instead of the entire production of *Contact!Unload* being staged, the script was adapted by George into a three-person performance piece called *UNLOAD*. *UNLOAD* invites the audience to connect with the actors and witness the courage they display as they confront trauma-related loss of a comrade and family member. It was performed three times by George and Phillip Lopresti.[1] I was able to dust off my guitar and provide the necessary soundtrack by playing live for this adaptation ... transitioning from visual artist to musician.

Note

1 The third actor for the Sydney production was Linden Wilkinson for two shows and Julie Hudspeth for the other.

7
Coming Home

Tim Laidler

THE 9/11 ATTACKS HAPPENED when I was a teenager in high school. Travelling on the school bus, a friend told me what had happened. I didn't know what to feel. I so badly wanted to believe it was not real. A year later I joined the Canadian Forces, and in 2008 deployed to Kandahar, Afghanistan. My mission overseas was to guard supply convoys, as our platoon travelled on roads continually attacked by the Taliban with suicide bombers and roadside bombs. I saw first-hand the desire the Afghan people had to feel safe, to go to school, and to improve their quality of life. This had a lasting impact, especially when I witnessed the collateral damage to civilians of failed bombing attacks by the Taliban.

Coming home to Canada, I was filled with purpose and gratitude that I survived. The good we did in Afghanistan was clear and I was so proud to have been part of the mission to rebuild the country. However, so many people in Canada still do not want to believe it was real. Barely anyone knew the purpose of our overseas mission, yet many like to share their opinions with someone in uniform. At social events, people would know I had been to Afghanistan yet they had no concept of what we did or what is was like for us coming home. The closest most Canadians can relate to is the experiences of their own families in the First and Second World Wars. This is often the starting point of conversations in an attempt at understanding, but in reality it is so different from what we experienced in Afghanistan. To explain the entire mission and how we were part of it is overwhelming for many veterans, myself included. It is easier to shut down any feelings that come up in conversation and listen politely to others talk about their family's service. After not talking about it for a while, it starts to feel less real. The tour overseas can feel like a dream, and your mind can play tricks on you and get you to question if you even went. So then the next time you talk about your tour, it is disconnected from any emotion, covered by some light humour.

Contact!Unload helps educate the public about what veterans have gone through and continue to go through now that they are home. As a veteran who took part in the art making (mural and Tribute Pole; see Chapter 6) and many of the performances, I find that it also reconnects veterans to their service and to one another. It helps us recall some of the emotions as we retell our own stories. By integrating the feelings we recall through the stories of serving, it also gives listeners a real point of connection. Not many people will be able to relate to the content of a war story, but almost everyone can relate to the feelings that come up during war – loss, pride, fear, or excitement. My participation in the art making and theatre, along with my current role as the chair of the board of the Veterans Transition Network, enables me to continue serving my country and fellow veterans through education initiatives and therapeutic opportunities.

8
Reconnaissance and Reclamation
Learning to Talk about the War

Anna Keefe

MY KNOWLEDGE OF WAR has always been limited. I grew up hearing fragments of stories about my grandfathers in the Second World War.

My mother's father fought with the US Navy in the Pacific as an anti-aircraft defence officer. Their destroyer, the USS *Melvin*, was in many successful campaigns and torpedoed and sank a Japanese battleship in the Battle of Leyte Gulf. They were being shot at constantly. My grandfather shot men whose faces he could see as they died. His leg caught fire. Many men he served with were so desperate for alcohol they made it from boot polish. But it wasn't all horror. They had a dog on the boat named Merciless Melvin. They convinced the captain to let them form a band to boost morale, and bought their instruments at a music shop in Honolulu. Fifty years later, my grandfather hosted exchange students from Japan and went to Japan in friendship to compete in the Senior Olympics.

But mostly he didn't like to talk about the war.

My father's father enlisted with the Canadian Armed Forces shortly before his eighteenth birthday. He began his service patrolling the coast of Newfoundland and playing hockey for the West Nova Scotia Regiment. He was trained as an officer and was sent to Sicily. He later landed on the toe of the Italian boot at Reggio. The Italians surrendered; the Germans left minefields in their path as they retreated. He was sent on a reconnaissance mission with three other men who all got shot by a sniper, and he expected to be next, but no shots came. My grandfather then walked up the middle of the deserted town of Potenza alone, the shutters creaking. He saw one of his own tanks and ran towards it waving, but it rolled over a mine and exploded. He woke up in a hospital in North Africa with a concussion and deaf in one ear. They patched him up and sent him back into many battles. He got malaria, his best friend was killed, he was hit by a motorcycle, and he finally came home to his wife and three-year-old child. Fifty years later, he returned to Italy, walked the cemeteries, and found the tombstones of so many people he had known.

But mostly he didn't like to talk about the war.

I heard some of these stories directly, but many second-hand from other family members, usually told with a mixture of pride and disbelief. In school, the World Wars were spoken of as necessary and noble at Remembrance Day assemblies. We always came prepared with our construction paper poppies and recitations of John McCrae's "In Flanders Fields":

> We are the dead. Short days ago
> We lived, felt dawn, saw sunset glow,
> Loved and were loved,[1]

Now I hear about war on the news – body counts, counter-terrorism, exit strategies. I hear about peace talks and ceasefires and hope for the best, vaguely worried, thoroughly detached. My sense of war has always been historical, academic, hypothetical, other-worldly. Many Canadians have the privilege of viewing war as abstract, but for others who serve in the armed forces and those who support them, war and its impacts are very real.

Contact!Unload was already well underway when I received an offer to get involved. My interests in arts education and trauma-informed practice dovetailed with the project. As a PhD student in Education at the University of British Columbia, I was deeply immersed in theories of teaching and learning, and was finally getting used to some of the norms and structures that both propelled and limited my work as a graduate student. Walking into the rehearsal space for the first time, I felt an awakening as I was reintroduced to the possibilities of emotionally and physically charged work. I noticed how present and communicative the veterans and team were. I realized that this was a space where academic norms were being resisted; where movement, expression, and relationships were respected as tools of inquiry. There was no tacit pressure to contain these aspects of my engagement with the world, or to present myself as intellectual by performing detachment and restraint.

I noticed how the veterans and facilitators watched for signs that they needed to offer each other encouragement, challenge, or time apart (see Figure 10). I noticed both a gravity and a freedom in the way people were expressing themselves, a collective effort to tell the story well. At first, I felt out of place, wondering if I was intruding on a deeply personal process, but I quickly felt welcomed and included. The veterans and facilitators checked in on me, shared personal stories and reflections on the work, and invited me to participate in their meals. They encouraged my input and helped me to understand the process as reciprocal, so that they were also helping me to learn and heal. During rehearsals I

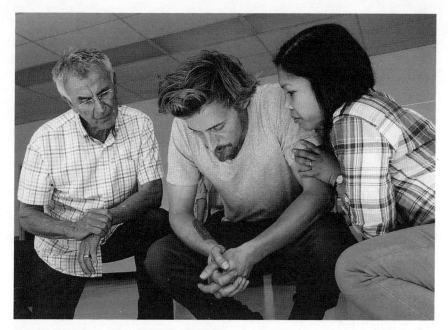

Figure 10 Marv Westwood (left) and JS Valdez (right) offering support to Tim Garthside (centre) during a rehearsal | Photo by Karen Forsyth; used with permission.

offered my help, my presence, and my growing understanding of the experiences of these veterans returning from war. I was also there to support the cast and crew during the three initial performances of *Contact!Unload,* where the magnitude of this project and its impact became apparent. I saw the intensity of the preparation and solidarity back stage, the audience affirmation and emotional resonance, and the relief and celebration. I too was caught up in the hope, as one veteran expressed, that the performance would reach at least one person who needed reassurance and inspiration to reach out for help. I came to see my role within the project as that of an observer, assistant, witness, and friend. I respect how this project used the power of art to navigate complexity, how partnerships allowed for generative risk-taking, and how telling a story of vulnerability and healing changed us all.

The arts have a powerful ability to deal with ambiguity and complexity by distilling life down to its most human and experiential elements. Through observation of the creative process of the *Contact!Unload* project, I saw how multiple voices and experiences, disparate opinions and realities, could be brought together into a cohesive whole. Every experience of war and return is different, and the piece of theatre was created in ways that did not attempt to dissolve those distinctions, but also linked everything with shared themes of mutual support and healing. Where one veteran was coping with post-traumatic stress and anxiety, another was missing the meaning and adrenaline that had characterized his experiences in combat. What a relief to pause before launching into political or moralistic deliberations of what should be; to pause for a moment to engage fully with the lived experiences of these men. I came to know the impacts of war and the chaos it has caused in their lives, but simultaneously grew to recognize their commitment to their military work and to each other. I came to understand their emotional and relational experiences of trying to rebuild their lives, their reclamation of love, their reckoning with ways they had wronged or been wronged, their ability to hold their involvement in war as both important and, at times, flawed. The sketches of each of my grandfathers at war began to take bolder shape and colour. The silences between their stories began to fill with the hum that ongoing survival sounds like.

During rehearsals, I remember standing in for a veteran who had become overwhelmed by the memory he was re-enacting. I read his lines in the scene while he took a walk with his counsellor. Telling his story, in his words, carrying it in my body as I moved across the stage, was profoundly moving. I became engaged at a new level with his trauma and resiliency. I was shaken out of academic forms of cognitive processing that I was being conditioned to accept as a graduate student – forms that too often skip into categorization and critique, that too often pass off disciplinary righteousness as rigour. Through my involvement with *Contact!Unload*, I became immersed in both a new area of knowledge and a new way of knowing. I could have easily applied modes of thinking that would lead me to distance myself by deconstructing the systemic injustices that lead to global conflict. Instead, I learned to find wholeness in contradiction and beauty in disarray and determination; I learned to sit with the discomfort of human complexity and agency. Learning through this process has inspired me to research in ways that locate and explore the lived experiences of participants, and to centre their realities in any broader analysis. Through this arts-based inquiry into life after combat, I found entry points into the complexity, and came to know war as real.

This project was ambitious and depended upon a positive orientation towards risk-taking and intentional engagement with difficulty. It was this urgent willingness to confront unresolved trauma, and to do so in new and innovative ways, that shocked me most. Were they not afraid that this bold truth seeking would be too much for the veterans or the audience? Were they not experimenting in ways that gave up control and certainty? I believe this generative risk-taking was possible because of the quality of the collaborative partnerships that sustained the project, and because of the courage and leadership of the veterans themselves. The University of British Columbia Department of Language and Literacy Education and Department of Educational and Counselling Psychology, and Special Education worked together to support the veterans and to follow their example of fearlessness. Each member of the team brought personal strengths and intentions as well as goals and sensibilities from within their disciplines/institutions. From the language and literacy contributors came knowledge of storytelling and theatre techniques; from the counselling contributors came knowledge of guiding clients through therapeutic re-enactment and potential triggers; from the veterans came experience with working under pressure and working as a team. Watching them at work, I wondered about the skills my grandfathers had brought back from the war, and about who had stepped up to support them as they took risks to seek and demonstrate resiliency.

I saw all members of this collaboration bring humility and willingness to learn, flexibility with roles and responsibilities, and attentiveness to relationships and communication. Many scenes were organized so that veterans could act alongside a counsellor and receive cues to help them stay grounded in moments of intensity during both rehearsals and performance. Tim Garthside described how rewarding it was to be in a space that allowed and required him to express a full range of emotions, to yell, to release those feelings he was trying to escape or contain. The director helped him do that in the most truthful and impactful way possible while the counsellors kept it safe and productive. By collaborating, we were able to support one another in working towards healing and raising public awareness by bringing the story to a broader audience.

This project was transformational for me and, I believe, for many participants and audience members as well. There was one monologue about connecting as a "band of brothers" that struck me as particularly true.[2] I recognized the feeling of loss Dale, the veteran, was describing when he shared a collective experience of hardship with his team and the fact that he had to leave them behind. I wept without expecting to. Dale sat with me and supported me in my moment of surprise emotion. He told me it was okay to take a break, to learn other things, to heal, and then go back to the work. We sat in the dark theatre and I was able to see myself. I was also able to see my grandfathers more clearly, and to wonder about the healing they had been offered or denied.

This is the beauty of theatre, and of this project in particular; we all had roles to maintain, but we were also equal in ways that let our shared humanity come to the surface. These veterans returned from the edge of an extreme reality to tell a story of what it means to be human. They returned from places of chaos and tenuous hope and brought back something valuable for each of us. What does it look like to not be okay? What does it look like to face that with courage and candid stories and hard work? Their gift was not just to other veterans but to every audience member who has known pain or pretended to be all right when they are not. We were invited first, and specifically, to see the reality of war and the road to recovery. We were invited second, and more generally, to witness what it looks like to seek mental and emotional wellness. The veterans told stories of healing as an uncertain journey. They told these stories with a generosity of spirit and compassion. They removed the shame and lifted up the everyday work of healing to show its texture and its likeness to our own faltering steps in moments of darkness.

My grandfathers didn't often talk to me about the war. But I remember now they had life-long friendships with other veterans. One sought peace years after the war in gestures of friendship with the Japanese, the other by paying his respects at the graves of those lost in battle in Italy. What was their journey towards healing in the years between? Through my involvement in this collaboration, I came to know war as real; I came to know risk as generative and collaboration as essential; I came to know myself. I traversed time and space to link this experience with the experiences of my grandfathers as veterans, and got to know them a little more.

Notes

1 J. McCrae and A. Macphail, *In Flanders Fields and Other Poems* (Toronto: W. Briggs, 1919), 3.

2 See Moment 19 in the Annotated Playscript in this volume.

9

Impact on Veteran Performers

George Belliveau, Blair McLean, and Christopher Cook

THIS CHAPTER SEEKS TO better understand *how* and *why* engaging in theatre making might yield positive therapeutic results for veterans who have experienced trauma and the civilians who supported them in the performance. To do so, we examine multiple data sources, including individual interviews with the veterans involved in developing and performing in the project, as well as debriefing sessions with veterans and civilian members of *Contact!Unload*.

Six male veterans – Chuck MacKinnon, Tim Garthside, Warren Geraghty, Dale Hamilton, Luke Bokenfohr, and Stephen Clews – agreed to provide us with insights regarding their experience in this theatre project, and participated in the individual interviews.[1] Four were Canadian Forces veterans and two served in militaries from other countries. Four of the six reported dealing with some form of military-related trauma. All six veteran participants successfully completed the Veterans Transition Program (VTP) prior to taking part in *Contact!Unload*. Four of the veterans participated in the devising and creation of the project during the initial phase in the winter/spring of 2015. All six veterans performed in the play in one or more of its iterations. We interviewed each participant individually with set questions for between thirty and forty-five minutes.

After the first two iterations of the play (April 2015 and November 2016), moderated post-production group debrief sessions were held with performing veterans and two civilian members of the cast and creative team. These sessions were over two hours in length and were facilitated by Dr. Marv Westwood. All of the interviews and debriefing sessions were video-recorded.

Process and Analysis

The first step in analyzing the collected data was to transcribe approximately three hours of interviews and five hours of debriefing sessions. Participants' bodies and gestures on the video recordings were also coded for analysis. We viewed the data through the lenses of Gestalt, drama, and sensorimotor therapy.

These therapies inform the action-based core of VTP therapeutic work, and helped the veterans lay the groundwork for participation in this theatre project. We utilized these three perspectives as we searched the transcripts for markers of therapeutic significance, including instances in which veterans noted their physical experience and shared their inner world, including emotionality, their stories about relationships and social connection, or meaningful events over the course of the production.

We also looked closely for anything they noticed that had changed for them personally between the time the theatre initiative began and ended. In the analysis, we separated all veteran self-reporting that referenced their personal experience of *Contact!Unload* from other conversation and banter, leaving approximately two and a half hours of interviews forming the narrative data pool from which we distilled the insights below.

Insights from the Data

Motivations

Some veterans were motivated to take part in the play based on their interest in the theatre, while hoping their participation might be of therapeutic benefit to them. Others expressed diverse motivations including educating the public, influencing government policy, informing fellow veterans about mental health, telling their war and transition stories to family and friends for the first time, and recruiting veterans in need of treatment to the VTP. Many of the reasons veterans gave for participation were externally focused, viewing taking part as a form of "service," with an emphasis on giving back to other veterans:

> CHUCK: Hopefully we'd make a difference ... [to] one young solider ... I wanted one vet. I would have been happy with that.

Civilians expressed being drawn to the project for similarly altruistic reasons – to make a difference. It is clear that most participants were not there for therapy per se; however, in unanticipated ways the theatre experience offered a strong therapeutic element fostering the personal change reported in the interviews and debriefs.

Unwelcome Change

Not all changes veterans underwent during the theatre process were comfortable, at least in the short term. Two of the veterans report becoming more consciously aware of past traumas:

CHUCK: Other things in my life are coming back up that I haven't thought about, people dying in emergency rooms and motor vehicle accidents, which is the other part of my life, and it's like fuck, that stuff I haven't thought about.

WARREN: The other side of it, um, is the awakening of all these old emotions ... Memories and emotions you know and ... also my service. ... Stuff that I don't want to remember.

Chuck and Tim speak further about an incursion of dreams and sleep disturbances:

TIM: I'm going to say I am in a better place even though I don't feel like it now, just because I'm so tired. I haven't been sleeping ... my dreams just wake me up. There's nights where I don't have nightmares, I just have really vivid dreams ... in my experience what happens when you're okay is that more things that need to be dealt with, um, just spring up. You can handle more so you get more.

CHUCK: The fucking dreaming started for me again. I get, I don't remember my dreams ... It drove me crazy, to the point where I thought I was going crazy. Now I'm just like, ah, fuck, not again, okay.

From a Gestalt perspective, change processes are non-linear, and discomfort may or may not indicate a setback.[2] Both Chuck and Tim speak to how, despite their discomfort, they noticed that they are moving forward, hinting at their increased capacity to tolerate and work with material from past trauma.

Embodied Trauma

In sensorimotor psychotherapy, embodied trauma is attributed to unfinished business in the body and the brain because of thwarted action during a traumatic experience, during which a person's attempt to defend himself or herself in the face of annihilation (real or imagined) proves ineffective.[3] Incomplete action becomes unfinished business because a part of the person is always trying to complete the action in an attempt to prevent the trauma. Tim, a former army signaller, describes his headset as a "cage" in *Contact!Unload*.[4] Through the headset, he was exposed to the voices of soldiers in distress that he could neither block out nor do anything to help aside from relaying their position and status to his officers. In Tim's interview, he tells how it felt to block his ears with his hands during the play:

TIM: What my body wants to do when that scream happens, when the gunfire happens, is to throw ... my hands over my ears and curl up in a ball, and so I did that and it felt good to be able to do that, to just, to do it.[5]

This passage is striking because Tim describes noticing he is triggered and acting on it. In *Contact!Unload*, he throws up his hands to protect himself, rather than suppressing the urge as he must do when he is triggered in public. The action is significant, given the nature of Tim's trauma. In this case, he shuts out the loud noises of screaming and gunfire in the play, while simultaneously completing the incomplete action of shutting out the sounds from his signaller's headset in the past. Pat Ogden and Janina Fisher argue that addressing thwarted self-protective attempts using defensive actions can help integrate trauma and empower individuals by enabling them to rebuild implicit trust in their defensive responses.[6] It is significant that Tim emphasizes this action in his narrative because a focal point of therapeutic change is embodied emotional experiencing and release, and the relief felt afterward. Before his dramatic change experience onstage, Tim recalls reporting to JS Valdez, a dramatherapist and assistant director of the play:

TIM: I voiced to her how uncomfortable I was in my body, like I just, I just felt awkward, I didn't know what to do with my body, didn't know where to put my hands.

Tim goes on to describe how Valdez validated his action impulses and encouraged him to give himself permission to notice what his body wanted to do and to experiment with various movements. Tim talks about how this permission allowed him to act authentically in the moment and release pent-up actions and emotions. This fits with the concepts of *embodiment* and *play* in the dramatherapy literature.[7] Using her training, Valdez helped Tim to explore the ways his body, trauma experience, and impulses for self-preservation were entwined, working towards congruence between his impulses and a concrete physical gesture (see Figure 10 in Chapter 8). She facilitated permission to experiment and play with various movements, some of which resonated with him strongly. Through this, Tim reports that connection between the play's content and his inner experience emerged.

Tim is adamant that, for him, change did not occur consciously while performing; instead he felt the change in his body and in the here and now:

TIM: There's no cognition. I wasn't thinking, it's just being ... there was no
thinking at all. It was purely being present in the moment and living those
experiences that are my, my story, living those exact moments as I do,
as I did.

Tim describes experiencing himself more fully in the moment, which is commensurate with Gestalt change theory. Like sensorimotor psychotherapy and dramatherapy, Gestalt therapy emphasizes the full experience of the self in the present as a vehicle for personal change.[8] Past trauma experiences must be "unloaded" and processed, as demonstrated in the therapeutic enactment (TE) scene in *Contact!Unload,* or they may become unfinished business.[9] Unfinished business is like a thorn in the side, demanding attention, steadily gaining power until the client's life becomes markedly impacted by preoccupation, compulsive behaviour, wariness, oppressive energy, and self-defeating behaviour.[10] Tim's words suggest that performing in *Contact!Unload* furthered the work he had begun through TE, as he speaks of a visceral embodied awareness in the here and now:

TIM: I felt like more of a conduit than anything. That just, the, the experience
was kind of just flowing through me ... I'm just in, in the flow. And that's
what I mean when I say I felt like a conduit.

His description of flow aligns with the Gestalt notion of tapping into the awareness continuum, an in-the-moment experiencing of whatever is most pertinent for an individual's growth and change.[11] Allowing his experience to flow through him, Tim appears to create a new body memory that might help him better cope with embodied trauma:

TIM: Having the experience of just letting it flow through me has allowed me
to realize that it can flow through me and when things are overpowering,
they're overpowering but I don't need to stay stuck in it.

Along with the flow, Tim reports physical and energetic experiences in his body:

TIM: Every cell in my body was vibrating, and not like I'm cold shaking but
like, almost imperceptible but like, my clothes were, I was vibrating.

Vibration may be an indicator of change for Tim, and certainly of movement. Tim's heightened awareness of it loads this sensation with meaning. It is also clear that the vibration experience is non-cognitive and occurring within the body, which may help to pinpoint the location of change. This phenomenon does not appear in the literature that the authors reviewed for this study.

Thawing Out

Over the course of engaging with *Contact!Unload,* the veterans paired action with emotional expression. As we witnessed the development process and closely examined the interviews and debriefing sessions, there was a clear display of emotion in their facial expressions, body movements, and postures while participating in the play. The data reveal examples that help us better understand how participating in theatre contributed to personal change, beginning with Tim's description of the personal cost of pent-up emotion:

> TIM: I've never been able to, uh, authentically embody emotion, even with, like, the VTP, with all of that stuff, it's always talking ... and whatever I am not letting out gets repressed and becomes anxiety ... I just was reflecting what was going on but not releasing anything.

In the play, Tim gained new awareness and granted himself permission to let the emotion go:

> TIM: It was okay to embody the emotion. I didn't know I needed the permission. I didn't have awareness around the fact that I had never embodied it.

Then came a dramatic shift with the outpouring of emotion, like a dam bursting, during Tim's "rant" onstage:[12]

> TIM: I didn't have to think about my lines, I didn't think, I wasn't thinking at all. It just kind of came out ... It was like I was a fuckin' emotion, an emotional beacon. I just had that emotional energy radiating out of every pore.

And the result:

> TIM: I felt, uh, lighter. And I attribute that to just not holding anything, any emotion ... it's easier to speak my truth and it's easier to live my truth because embodying the emotion is just as important as speaking the emotion.

Tim experienced a profound change in himself related to emotional release. This might be partially explained by the dramatherapy concept of catharsis: the expression or release of emotions resulting in a sudden shift in perception and the acquisition of insight.[13] As Tim explains, his perceptual shift was one of embodying emotion, of connecting the outpouring of emotion to the physical experience of the body, as opposed to talking about emotions. Giving permission to the impulse to release emotion in connection with the body facilitates access to implicit memories, and transformative knowledge is accrued by tapping into a felt sense of the wisdom of the body.[14] In Tim's case, the performance of long-dormant actions, culminating in emotional and physical expression, seems to have fostered a profound change and enabled him to process and integrate implicit memories related to his trauma.

Nobody Told Me I Was a Monster

For Tim, the compassionate witnessing of the audience during the public presentations of *Contact!Unload* was transformational, deepening and solidifying a change he had begun to make during his time in the VTP. This change involved rewriting the core belief "I am a monster" scrawled on his soul the instant he learned he had inadvertently ordered the death of an allied informant in Afghanistan. Tim's lived experience of relaying the go-ahead to eliminate someone perceived as an enemy during a firefight is a key scene in *Contact!Unload*.[15] In this scene, audiences witness Tim trying to save injured Canadian soldiers lying on the ground. Through radio interaction, he was led to believe that an informant was an enemy target that needed to be eliminated before the wounded could be rescued.

In the VTP, Tim accessed his trauma through his body and began to internalize empathy and forgiveness from other group members, fellow veterans, who acknowledged how terrible Tim's situation was without labelling him as a terrible person. This was the beginning of his healing process. The next step was taking in additional messages of acceptance, this time from civilians and family while he was physically activated during performances of *Contact!Unload*.

TIM: Nobody told me I was a monster. There was no negative anything. Everyone was thanking me ... along those lines of, of, that's brave, you're, thank you ...

In the case of Tim, a soldier experiencing alienation after serving his country, the audience witnesses and helps to bear responsibility, on behalf of all Canadian people, for the actions he regrets. The witnessing, and to a certain degree the acceptance and forgiveness of the audience, enables Tim to continue his healing process.

Never Alone: Social-Connectedness

On a few occasions, several veterans indicated that they would elect in an instant to go back overseas to fight. As researchers, we assumed that, given some of the participants' experiences of acute trauma, they would rather be anywhere but in a war zone. Later we learned that this could be partially explained by the loss of adrenaline-charged experiences, as depicted in the play, particularly in Moment 5. The veterans characterized the friendships they developed in service with feelings of absolute trust. Losing those relationships is extremely difficult and seems to play a significant role in veterans' difficult transitions back to civilian life. Dale describes the importance to him of social-connectedness in the military:

> DALE: You work and train alongside the same guys day in and day out and then on your time off you end up hanging out with the same guys, because they're your friends. It's a bond that, next to family, I can't think of anything that comes close.

An enormous challenge for those who come back is to replace this unique social-connectedness of the military community. Often veterans elect to spend time with other veterans, but, despite the hard work of organizations like the Canadian Legion, opportunities for veteran community building remain few and far between. *Contact!Unload,* similar to the group approach of the VTP, filled this gap for its participants, at least over the course of the months of the play's development and performances. Luke uses the metaphor of a "fire team" to describe his experience of bonding with the other veterans while performing *Contact!Unload:*

> LUKE: It's like, a fire team really, we're a fire team, right, which is a, which is your smallest, tightest group within the military ... You're digging the trench together. You're literally sleeping in a bivvy [sleeping bag] next to a guy, you know, back to back or whatever, you know, two guys on sentry, two guys sleeping ... it's the tightest bond you got.

The bond is particularly tight in a fire team because at any moment they could be under fire. This metaphor speaks to the unique combination in the play of fostering friendships, working hard to prepare for performances, and the

Impact on Veteran Performers 87

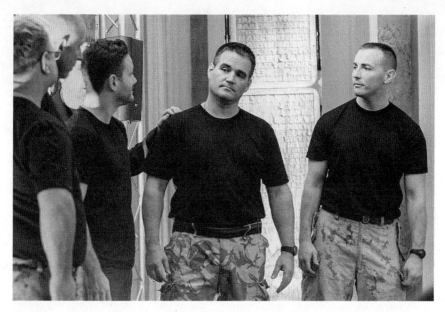

Figure 11 "It's like a fire team." Performing at Canada House. Left to right: Chuck MacKinnon, Mike Waterman, Luke Bokenfohr, and Stephen Clews | Photo by Blair McLean; used with permission.

adrenaline rush associated with performing in front of an audience. Without all these pieces, including time together, hard work, and nerves around the performance, the level of social-connectedness and purpose would likely not be as high. Stephen speaks to what having purpose with fellow veterans meant to him:

> STEPHEN: I was unhappy when I came back to Canada. I never really renewed that purpose that I had. What I enjoyed was having a purpose with people who are like-minded ... Everyone here [veterans and civilians] is exceptionally important to me ... This is one of those things that will stand out no matter what, and it's because of the people in this [play].

Stephen speaks about like-mindedness as if its presence is a fact. His certainty may partially be due to the unspoken bond that veterans share through a kind of club membership. The camaraderie between participants in this project was experienced rather than spoken. It was initiated through embodied empathy fostered by the group process and shared experience of play creation. Warren's experience is particularly congruent with this idea of new bond creation within the context of *Contact!Unload*. For him, acceptance was never a given:

WARREN: I'm not a Canadian veteran and I always felt like a bit of an intruder and I wasn't made to feel like that at all. It felt very, very awkward for me to be in at the beginning, very, very difficult. So I want to thank the veterans for accepting me ... They just accepted me with open arms and, uh, and drew me in, it was fantastic, a great feeling, and I'll always be, I'll always have that feeling, I'll always cherish these guys.

In this passage, Warren speaks explicitly about his experience of change. When he first met with our group, he saw himself as an outsider, and by naming this in the group, he alerted the other veterans to his inner experience. In turn, they empathized with and supported him in such a way that his feeling changed to one of inclusion.

The interview and debriefing data highlight how participation in *Contact!-Unload* helped to meet veterans' needs for social-connectedness. This echoes the larger unmet need for veterans in transition for social connection. It also begs the question of how new venues to help veterans connect in meaningful ways might be established. The project included a relatively long-term (four-month) development, rehearsal, and production format, in which veterans and civilians worked towards a shared goal, performing in a group in front of an audience. Another strength of theatre is that it may foster social connection between veterans and civilians in the community, particularly if it includes post-show discussions and social gatherings, as *Contact!Unload* attempted to do. This too facilitates veteran transition and integration by exposure between population groups that might not otherwise interact. Such communion between civilians and veterans may help veterans unlearn mistrust and learn that they do not have to restrict themselves to veterans' groups only.

Personal Mastery and Reconstruction of Identity
Theatre has the potential to develop a variety of important skills, including leadership, personal mastery, competence, and the expansion of identity through the development of trust in one's ability to create, collaborate, and perform.[16] Veterans who suffer from trauma often experience a significant barrier to such developmental growth. Chuck, who lives with post-traumatic stress (PTS), offers an example of theatre unlocking a door:

CHUCK: I had lost creativity. I had lost the, the want, the desire to be onstage. [VTP] brought it back and this [play] fostered it beyond my dreams. I just, years ago, dreamed that maybe one day I would be onstage and shit, there we were.

From his experience with the play, it seems that Chuck will take with him a new internal understanding of his capacity for creativity as well as his ability to perform onstage. Warren speaks to how performing increased his confidence in himself:

WARREN: It's given me that, a lot more confidence. You know you're up in front of people and speaking to people ... the performance anxiety died down ... and the confidence went way up.

Warren's newfound confidence is an indicator of personal and interpersonal mastery reinforced by his experience of standing in front of the audience and skillfully communicating. Theatre performance, in this case, is a form of behavioural rehearsal whereby participants practise communicating their authentic inner experiences to others in ways that might have been difficult in the past. The more Warren practised and was exposed to discomfort in the situation, the more his mind and body knew that he could do it again in the future. This led to an increase in confidence.

Dale suggests that sharing autobiographical stories of military-related trauma not only provided relief but increased his self-efficacy in processing these experiences:

DALE: Having these stories ... inside and not talking about them is, is poisonous, I think; it, it, um, it makes everything so much worse ... Writing about it – taking that experience and putting it onto paper, I find it's almost a dropping of baggage. It's an unburdening of that story. And then reading it to a group of strangers, um, it's possibly the best thing I've done ... for my own self.

In sharing his personal stories of trauma through writing and performance, Dale mastered a new resource for "dropping baggage." Rather than showing a veteran "poisoned" by holding trauma in, Dale's words suggest the construction of a new identity: a veteran capable of combating trauma with expression and storytelling.

Civilian Voices
The civilian participants' words also demonstrate significant personal change, and depict *Contact!Unload* as a means of relationship building between veterans and civilians as they work together to create theatre. Oliver expresses both a sense of having made a contribution and a greater empathic understanding of the traumas veterans face:

OLIVER: When George said his line from the play "now that was something," my brain automatically completed Tim's line: "Afghanistan was something and when I was there I was something" ... because, well, the script is pretty well engraved in my head after all those hours of rehearsal ... and I was briefly in Afghanistan for about five minutes over three nights. Those words came to mind because being part of this has been something ... something that I'm really proud to have been a part of ... and I feel like I contributed to a project that makes some sort of difference ... for the guys that came and told us after performances that they were going to look at getting counselling themselves ... for those family members that said they feel like they understand their loved ones better ... and for me and the members of my family that came to it ... we've gotten a better sense of a really important institution in our country, one for which people make sacrifices that go unappreciated.

Oliver briefly had an embodied understanding of what it might mean to be serving in Afghanistan during each performance. He also describes a "cathartic" release similar to those experienced by the veterans, in which raw emotional feeling gave way to a newfound sense of peace:

OLIVER: On closing night we had that sort of cathartic post-production session and I came away from that feeling quite raw ... and I haven't sort of woken up. I woke up that next morning and I felt a sense of something's changed. We've moved on a bit. I don't have a sense of sorrow. I have a sense of pride. I've had challenges in my life over the past couple of months and I've felt more relaxed over that past few weeks than I have in a year or two. This has been a wonderful thing to be a part of and it's made a difference for me and I'm confident it has made a difference for others.

Similarly, Mike speaks of being cathartically activated throughout the creation process, describing ongoing moments of emotional release:

MIKE: Being involved with the creation and performance of *Contact!Unload* has had a major impact on me and continues to do so. When I got involved, I did so because I knew it was for a good purpose but I don't think I realized the scope of the impact it would have on everyone involved. To see the veterans continue their service in another form, putting themselves out there in order to help others, has been inspiring. Growing close to the guys and seeing what they are doing every performance and knowing their purpose deeply, it's difficult not to lose it onstage. It took months of answering the question "What was it like working on this project?" to be able to answer without breaking down.

In seeing the veterans' dedication to the project, and watching them develop new theatre skills, Mike was motivated to make changes in his own life:

MIKE: Seeing the veterans dedicating themselves to a project that must be incredibly difficult at times with such drive, purpose, and confidence has made me want to do the same in all aspects of my life, which is a great gift. As Chuck and others have said on many occasions, as long as one veteran gets the help they may need, then the whole project has been worth it.

Discussion and Conclusion

We are aware that this chapter explores the change narratives of only a limited number of participants, and we therefore make no claims that our findings and insights are generalizable. However, two recent theatre-based projects briefly described in the Introduction found similar insights into release and change in veterans' narratives. Alison O'Connor describes the impact of a three-month project with veterans in Wales who brought difficult narratives of trauma in *Abandoned Brothers*.[17] The theatre initiative inspired the veterans and some of their family members to form "a support group, which meets every week. They run it themselves, have recruited more members ... [and have created] a place for healing and peace where a lot more stories will be told."[18] Linda Hassall and Michael Balfour similarly illustrate how veterans working on the Difficult Return project in Brisbane, Australia, reported that they were able to release some of their trauma and move forward in their lives in positive ways due to personal insights gained from the theatre project.[19]

This study suggests that therapy through theatre facilitates a multimodal change process making use of experiential, action-oriented, body-based, social, behavioural, developmental, narrative, and emotional mechanisms for change. But despite its tremendous therapeutic potential, the theatre remains underutilized by counsellors for various reasons, including confidentiality and ethical constraints, entrenched conventions such as talk-therapy, funding structures, and the unfamiliarity of many counsellors with play creation and the arts. *Contact!Unload* demonstrates a model of how a careful exploration of progressive therapeutic paradigms grounded in ethical practices and informed consent, combined with a collective play-creation process, may yield positive outcomes for participants.

Notes

This chapter is derived in part from G. Belliveau, C. Cook, B. McLean, and G.W. Lea, "Thawing Out: Therapy through Theatre with Canadian Military Veterans," *The Arts in Psychotherapy* 62 (2019): 45–51, https://doi.org/10.1016/j.aip.2018.11.001.

1 This research was approved by the University of British Columbia Behavioural Research Ethics Board #H15-00111. All participants wished to use their real names.

2 F.S. Perls, *Gestalt Therapy: Excitement and Growth in the Human Personality* (New York: Julian Press, 1951).

3 P. Ogden and J. Fisher, *Sensorimotor Psychotherapy: Interventions for Trauma and Attachment* (New York: W.W. Norton, 2015).

4 See Moment 21 in the Annotated Playscript in this volume.

5 This refers to Moment 21.

6 Ogden and Fisher, *Sensorimotor Psychotherapy*.

7 P. Jones, *Drama as Therapy: Theory, Practice and Research,* 2nd ed. (New York: Routledge, 2007).

8 Perls, *Gestalt Therapy*.

9 See Moment 21.

10 G. Corey, *Theory and Practice of Counseling and Psychotherapy,* 9th ed. (Belmont, CA: Brooks Cole, 2012).

11 L. Perls, "Concepts and Misconceptions of Gestalt Therapy," *Journal of Humanistic Psychology* 32, 3 (1992): 50–56, https://doi.org/10.1177/0022167892323004.

12 See Moment 16. In this rant, he shows his frustration over how civilians are unable to understand or comprehend struggles like the one he experienced during his service in Afghanistan.

13 J.L. Moreno, *The Essential Moreno: Writings on Psychodrama, Group Method, and Spontaneity* (New York: Springer, 1987).

14 M.J. Westwood and P. Wilensky, *Therapeutic Enactment: Restoring Vitality through Trauma Repair in Groups* (Vancouver: Group Action Press, 2005).

15 See Moment 21.

16 D. Beare and G. Belliveau, "Theatre for Positive Youth Development: A Development Model for Collaborative Play-Creating," *Applied Theatre Researcher/IDEA Journal* 8 (2007): 1–16.

17 A. O'Connor, "*Abandoned Brothers,* Life Story Theatre with Veterans and Their Families," *Arts and Health* 7, 2 (2015): 151–60, https://doi.org/10.1080/17533015.2015.1011177.

18 Ibid., 159.

19 L. Hassall and M. Balfour, "Transitioning Home: Research-Based Theatre with Returning Servicemen and Their Families," in *Research-Based Theatre: An Artistic Methodology,* ed. G. Belliveau and G.W. Lea, 103–16 (Bristol: Intellect, 2016); L. Hassall, *The Return* (unpublished script, 2014).

10

Holding on to the Script

Phillip Lopresti

> *Therapy, in a very real sense, is theatre. It's a dramatic event in which the story emerges from the interaction of embodied players, each affecting the other in a continuously unfolding dance.*
>
> – ARTHUR ROBERTS, THE DREAMER AND THE DREAM[1]

THE STORIES THAT EMERGED from the making and performing of *Contact!-Unload* resemble a process as collaborative and fluid as the one described by Arthur Roberts.[2] The moving scenes and dialogue of the play not only illustrate the struggles of military life but also set the stage for the surfacing of more nuanced issues that have eluded public awareness for decades. The materialization of the subject matter is facilitated by the collaborative playmaking process and is presented in the form of research-based theatre.[3] There are numerous therapeutic modalities at play within this process; however, within this chapter I will comment on four experiences related to healing within the context of *Contact!Unload:* a gender-informed approach to post-traumatic stress (PTS), tableaux, group processing, and audience presence. *Contact!Unload* worked from a gender-informed approach to PTS as it mobilized characteristics of theatre that were well aligned with the masculine ideals held by the veteran performers. Furthermore, the military's focus on the physical, as well as this performance's utilization of embodied experiences such as tableau development, contributed greatly to the success of the performance and the positive experience shared by the veteran and civilian performers. These movements were conducted in group settings, advancing the exercise's cultural congruency with the veterans and the resultant unearthing of new understandings. The genuineness of the performers' emotions served to draw in the audience, compelling them to listen assiduously and respond with their own truths. It is in this moment of exchange between performers and audience that another therapeutic component of the play is thought to reside.

In this chapter, I use my own involvement in *Contact!Unload* as well as literature about the arts and counselling to hold a conversation on how the two intersect to facilitate healing for post-traumatic stress injuries. I do this from the perspective of a participant as well as a student in counselling psychology. Furthermore, I incorporate my own experience of military service to draw attention to processes that exist in both theatre and the military. This chapter should be read as a commentary on some of the therapeutic elements of theatre present within *Contact!Unload,* and should not be considered as a complete or in-depth exploration of the vast and complex work found in collaborative playmaking and research-based theatre.

A Gender-Informed Understanding

An advantage I had when deciding to enlist with the Canadian Armed Forces (CAF) was that I possessed a significant understanding of the psychological risks associated with combat-related injuries. In particular, I understood how the military commodified masculinity and reinforced hegemonic ideals while unknowingly increasing the risk for perceived failure to uphold a masculine identity if injured.[4] Understanding the risk of how my self-perception of masculinity might change as a result of an injury, either physical or psychological, made me feel as though I was making a more informed decision to join. Unfortunately, this has not been the norm for all who have decided to agree to the unlimited liability of joining the army. To address this gap in people's understanding of gendered experiences of post-traumatic stress injuries, I begin this chapter with an overview of literature that has focused on how those who subscribe to traditional ideals of masculinity experience PTS, and later connect these ideals to theatrical performance. While the literature suggests that rates of PTS may be higher in women after traumatic incidents, PTS does not discriminate by gender, age, sexual orientation, or ethnicity.[5] Research does suggest, however, that the experience of PTS may differ across genders. While cisgender men tend to experience greater irritability, hypervigilance, amnesia, and substance use, cisgender women tend to experience more flashbacks and trauma recall, including reports of previous traumatic childhood histories.[6] Cisgender men's ways of experiencing PTS tend to be based on socially constructed hypermasculinized gender scripts.[7] These scripts encourage men to:

- be stoic and in control of themselves
- be able to manage emotions, especially those associated (or deemed associated) with being vulnerable
- be fearless and indestructible

- consider anger to be the only acceptable masculine emotion
- be competitive, achievement-oriented, and successful
- be strong and independent
- exemplify the opposite of any of the characteristics associated with either femininity or behaviours associated with same-sex attraction.[8]

It should be noted that individuals who do not identify as cisgender men (such as cisgender women and trans* individuals) who operate in hyper-masculinized environments such as the military may also follow these scripts.[9] Regardless of gender or orientation, these personnel tend to endorse higher levels of male gender role socialization related to military disciplinary culture.[10] This is a key factor that exacerbates how they experience stigma.[11] While the endorsement of traditional masculine ideals (e.g., being fearless, achievement-oriented, and competitive; valuing traits such as loyalty and self-reliance; and identifying themselves through their bodies) has many positive aspects, it is also associated with a host of problematic issues, such as poor self-esteem, reduced interpersonal intimacy, depression, and anxiety.[12] Those who endorse these ideals are often faced with gender role discrepancy strain, such that if they successfully subscribe to these unrealistic and contradictory masculine ideologies and then deviate from masculine norms, psychological strain follows as a result of a person's behaviour being inconsistent with socially prescribed norms.[13] When these gender role violations occur, the resulting strain can be experienced as overwhelmingly unpleasant, so that many compensate by adhering even more rigidly to traditional definitions of masculinity.[14] This is problematic; as a growing body of research suggests, there is a strong association between the degree to which individuals endorse traditional or dominant masculine ideologies and poor health behaviours. Avoidance of therapy is one of these behaviours. Many who choose to avoid therapy do so because it is perceived as an activity that involves disclosing weaknesses or problems, which, for many, is threatening to their strictly held masculine identities. Unfortunately, this avoidance may perpetuate further emotional isolation.[15] Having had no previous experience with theatre myself, I was quite shocked to learn just how physically and cognitively challenging performing could be. I was also surprised that rather than challenging my masculine identity, theatre appeared to enhance it.

How Theatre Is Hard

Although I can't speak to whether or not the other performers found performing as challenging as I did, an argument can be made for how the demands of performing are well aligned with masculine ideals. Besides the psychological challenges of theatre, performing also requires physical discipline and jurisdiction over one's body. To explore the physicality of theatre further, I shift the discussion to some of the embodied components of the collaborative playmaking process and research-based theatre that have contributed to the success of *Contact!Unload* as a medium for healing.

Tableaux

Throughout the development of *Contact!Unload,* tableaux were used as launching points for the development of monologues and scenes woven throughout the piece. George Belliveau describes a tableau as a "frozen image or picture with participants using their *bodies* to illustrate their meaning in a realistic or symbolic manner."[16] Rather than describing moments or experiences with words, tableaux focus on "just showing, [not] talking."[17] This is not unlike family sculpting – a technique used frequently in group and family counselling.[18] Family sculpting is employed to bypass intellectualization and defensiveness in order to reveal hidden aspects of the individual or system in which the individual holds membership.[19] Within theatre, moments of silence and discomfort can produce "strong images" and help the players discover "body language and internal dialogue" not otherwise accessible to them.[20] Likewise, within family sculpting, it is during moments of silence that some of the greatest revelations occur. The mandatory silence prevents family members from projecting blame onto the others and compels them to carry out an internal dialogue promoting self-exploration and growth.[21] Relatedly, the result of having the veterans engage in these "embodied experiences" was the revelation of "new understandings and emotional responses" not previously shared.[22]

Based on my own military experience, the success of embodied process in this project is not surprising. Military culture prides itself on physical prowess and continuously seeks to push the human body beyond what was previously thought possible. During training exercises, it quickly became apparent that I was indeed capable of much more than I had previously thought possible. Although I did not immediately appreciate the twenty-kilometre forced marches or deliberate sleep deprivation, I did come to be more attuned to my body and what it was capable of. In combat training, a tremendous amount of stress is placed on individuals, so much so that the body reverts to autonomic processes embedded in the subconscious.[23] Combat instructors capitalize on this by pushing candidates beyond the point of intellectualization, and then embedding routine and procedure to allow soldiers to remain combat-effective under severe duress. However, just as routine can be stored in the body, so can trauma. Marv Westwood speaks to the importance of movement in therapy, particularly for those who have suffered a traumatic event, as a way to free traumatic experiences stored in the body.[24] It may be, then, that when veterans were engaged in activities involving movement and body awareness, previously suppressed cognitions and emotions were liberated. In this way, tableaux may make space for the subconscious to emerge and shift story in directions not originally intended.

Group

When working with individuals living with PTS, it is critical to understand how their symptoms contribute to increasingly pervasive social isolation. Re-experiencing symptoms, such as intrusive thoughts of the traumatic event (especially surrounding recurring reminders of the trauma), can isolate individuals by limiting their drive to engage outside of perceived "safe" boundaries.[25] Hyperarousal symptoms, such as constant hypervigilance and irritable or angry outbursts, can exacerbate already strained relationships, with traumatized individuals feeling that they are beyond assistance and alone in their suffering. Finally, emotional avoidance and numbing symptoms, such as disconnection and detachment from loved ones and loss of interest in previously enjoyed activities, amplify self-isolating behaviours as it is often easier to avoid triggers than attempt to deal with them.[26]

In light of these challenges, group counselling can provide a safe setting that encourages members to share and take risks, which enables them to participate in their own healing process.[27] It has also been suggested that group therapy can be one way to prevent overwhelming emotional distress through safe, structured emotional release.[28] Group process can also correct distorted thinking and reduce feelings of shame and guilt through normalization of experience.[29] Research has also shown that individual therapy may not improve interpersonal difficulties that result from trauma; thus, group therapy may be a more effective treatment setting for individuals living with PTS.[30] As Marianne Cory and colleagues have aptly put it, "individuals are wounded in relationships and can heal in relationships."[31]

Time and cost-effectiveness are also important factors to consider, especially when trying to meet the needs of an underserved population.[32] While it may seem intuitive that these may increase accessibility of help for any population, it is particularly important to consider them when working with a group such as veterans, who may already be resistant to help seeking.[33] Whether individuals who need help are hindered by social factors such as those discussed earlier in this chapter, or by lack of awareness of the options available, getting help must be kept as simple as possible to ensure that they are not left in the dark for too long, as the damage can be irreversible. Group therapy is indeed one way to serve more people in need while minimizing the cost to them and their providers.

In line with these principles of group therapy, during the initial development of *Contact!Unload*, a large amount of time was dedicated to group check-ins, where members of the cast and development team took time to share their personal stories. This allowed the group to develop a sense of "trust and community."[34] The sense of safety resulting from time spent on this stage of group process most likely contributed to the success of the embodied experiences, mentioned at the beginning of this chapter, and their ability to surface "deep emotional responses."[35] This may be the case because in order to explore and discuss one's feelings, an activity not typically engaged in by men, any fear of judgment or ridicule must be absent.[36] Furthermore, pausing after these moments of self-disclosure and allowing the group to process the content together provided group members with an opportunity to support each other, increasing their own feelings of self-efficacy.[37]

Audience Impact on Healing

As part of his master's thesis at the University of British Columbia, Blair McLean followed the experience of six of the veterans who performed in *Contact!Unload* and observed how the empathic witnessing of the audience was transformative for the veterans and contributed to advancements over their previous therapeutic experiences.[38] George Belliveau supports this by suggesting that when the veterans share their stories, the weight of the emotional baggage being carried by the individual is lessened, and a sense of being understood results from being publicly "witnessed by others."[39] Although he and Jennica Nichols do not focus on the therapeutic benefits of audience presence for the veterans, they do point to the ability of theatre to provide "humanity and emotional connection" that might not have otherwise been possible.[40] It is through this shared emotional experience of the veterans and audience members that cathartic witnessing is able to take place. As within group work, the emotional responses from the audience, both direct and indirect, can act as relational feedback, fostering a sense of connectedness and feelings of being understood.[41] This new sense of being understood is then internalized and results in the development of increased self-esteem such that the individual feels more congruent with how they would like to feel about themselves.[42]

It is not possible, however, to fully attribute the positive outcomes associated with *Contact!Unload* to audience presence. Within narrative therapy, the deconstruction of problematic narratives and re-storying of them is a common practice that can yield positive results for clients suffering psychological ailments such as major depressive disorder.[43] Moreover, the delivery of narrative therapy is typically done in one-on-one sessions rather than in groups, further suggesting that audience presence may not be necessary to evoke the therapeutic change.[44] These conflicting findings suggest that more work is needed to explore how the experiences of the veteran performers in projects such as *Contact!Unload* are shaped by audience presence.

Conclusion

Throughout this chapter, I have drawn attention to four critical components of the collaborative playmaking process in the development and delivery of *Contact!Unload*. The first was tableaux development as an embodied experience. This also acted as a foundation to the second factor, working in a gender-informed manner, which allowed for the surfacing of veterans' hidden emotions that until then remained at a subconscious level. Tableaux seemed to act as a catalyst to move past the unconscious processes that served as gatekeepers to authentic emotional disclosure. What ultimately made it safe to disclose these deeply personal and often shameful thoughts were the group dynamics present within the dramatic work, which constituted the third critical factor. Finally, the fourth factor, which possibly solidified the therapeutic work that had already taken place in the development of the performance piece was the empathic witnessing of the audience. Through this exchange of emotion between players and audience members, it is possible that performers were able to integrate their wounds as they witnessed the hundreds of audience members embracing their stories with great care and compassion. The work that took place in this project was indeed profound and should be further explored in order to better understand how the arts and storytelling enable psychological healing for post-traumatic stress.

Notes

1 A. Roberts, "Theatre and Therapy," in *The Dreamer and the Dream: Essays and Reflections on Gestalt Therapy*, by Rainette Eden Fantz and Arthur Roberts (New York: Routledge, 1998), 15.

2 Ibid.

3 G. Belliveau and G.W. Lea, eds., *Research-Based Theatre: An Artistic Methodology* (Bristol: Intellect, 2016).

4 D.M. Shields, D. Kuhl, and M.J. Westwood, "Abject Masculinity and the Military: Articulating a Fulcrum of Struggle and Change," *Psychology of Men and Masculinity* 18, 3 (2017): 215–25, https://doi.org/10.1037/men0000114.

5 American Psychiatric Association, *Diagnostic and Statistical Manual of Mental Disorders*, 5th ed. (Washington, DC: American Psychiatric Association, 2013); T.J. Shaffer, "A

Comparison of Firefighters and Police Officers: The Influence of Gender and Relationship Status," *Adultspan Journal* 9, 1 (2010): 36–49; D. Silove, J.R. Baker, M. Mohsin, M. Teesson, et al., "The Contribution of Gender-Based Violence and Network Trauma to Gender Differences in Post-Traumatic Stress Disorder," *PLOS One* 12, 2 (2017): 1–12.

6   C.C. Lee, ed., *Multicultural Issues in Counseling: New Approaches to Diversity* (Hoboken, NJ: John Wiley and Sons, 2014).

7   Ibid.

8   Ibid., 302.

9   Here, I use "trans*" to encompass individuals who do not identify as cisgender (transgender, genderqueer, non-binary, two-spirit, and others).

10 R. Hinojosa, "Doing Hegemony: Military, Men, and Constructing a Hegemonic Masculinity," *Journal of Men's Studies* 18, 2 (2010): 179–94.

11 C.W. Hoge, C.A. Castro, S.C. Messer, D. McGurk, et al., "Combat Duty in Iraq and Afghanistan, Mental Health Problems, and Barriers to Care," *New England Journal of Medicine* 351, 1 (2004): 13–22.

12 J. Mahalik, G.E. Good, and M. Englar-Carlson, "Masculinity Scripts, Presenting Concerns and Help-Seeking: Implications for Practice and Training," *Professional Psychology: Research and Practice* 34 (2003): 123–31.

13 C.M. Rummell and R.F. Levant, "Masculine Gender Role Discrepancy Strain and Self-Esteem," *Psychology of Men and Masculinity* 15, 4 (2014): 419–26, https://doi.org/10.1037/a0035304.

14 J.H. Pleck, *The Myth of Masculinity* (Cambridge, MA: MIT Press, 1981).

15 W.H. Courtenay, "Constructions of Masculinity and Their Influence on Men's Wellbeing: A Theory of Gender and Health," *Social Science and Medicine* 50, 10 (2000): 1385–1401.

16 G. Belliveau, "Engaging in Drama: Using Arts-Based Research to Explore a Social Justice Project in Teacher Education," *International Journal of Education and the Arts* 7, 5 (2006): 4, http://www.ijea.org/v7n5/v7n5.pdf.

17 Ibid.

18 P. Papp, O. Silverstein, and E. Carter, "Family Sculpting in Preventive Work with 'Well Families,'" *Family Process* 12, 2 (1973): 197–212, https://doi.org/10.1111/j.1545-5300.1973.00197.x.

19 Ibid.

20 Belliveau, "Engaging in Drama," 5.

21 Papp, Silverstein, and Carter, "Family Sculpting in Preventive Work."

22 G. Belliveau, "Theatre with Veterans: Transition and Recovery," *Journal of Applied Arts and Health* 8, 2 (2017): 258.

23 D. Buss, *Evolutionary Psychology,* 5th ed. (Boston: Pearson, 2015).

24 M.J. Westwood, "The Veterans Transition Program: Therapeutic Enactment in Action," *Educational Insights* 13, 2 (2009), http://einsights.ogpr.educ.ubc.ca/v13n02/articles/westwood/index.html.

25 A.L. Chapman, K.L. Gratz, and M.T. Tull, *The Dialectical Behavior Therapy Skills Workbook for Anxiety: Breaking Free from Worry, Panic, PTSD and Other Anxiety Symptoms* (Oakland, CA: New Harbinger, 2011).

26 Ibid.

27 M.S. Corey, G. Corey, and C. Corey, *Groups: Process and Practice,* 9th ed. (Belmont, CA: Brooks/Cole, 2014).

28 V. Rozynko and H.E. Dondershine, "Trauma Focus Group Therapy for Vietnam Veterans with PTSD," *Psychotherapy: Theory, Research, Practice, Training* 28, 1 (1991): 157–61.

29 Ibid.

30 S.M. Glynn, S. Eth, E.T. Randolph, D.W. Foy, et al., "A Test of Behavioral Family Therapy to Augment Exposure for Combat-Related Posttraumatic Stress Disorder," *Journal of Consulting and Clinical Psychology* 67, 2 (1999): 243–51.

31 Corey, Corey, and Corey, *Groups*, 3.

32 R.H. Klein and V.L. Schermer, eds., *Group Psychotherapy for Psychological Trauma* (New York: Guilford Press, 2000).

33 Courtenay, "Constructions of Masculinity."

34 Belliveau, "Theatre with Veterans," 258.

35 Ibid.

36 Rummell and Levant, "Masculine Gender Role Discrepancy Strain and Self-Esteem."

37 Westwood, "The Veterans Transition Program."

38 B.W. McLean, "*Contact!Unload*: A Narrative Study and Filmic Exploration of Veterans Performing Stories of War and Transition" (master's thesis, University of British Columbia, 2017), https://doi.org/10.14288/1.0343358.

39 Belliveau, "Theatre with Veterans," 259.

40 G. Belliveau and J. Nichols, "Audience Responses to *Contact!Unload*: A Research-Based Play about Returning Military Veterans," *Journal of Cognitive Psychology: Arts and Humanity* 4, 1 (2017): 6.

41 M.J. Westwood, H. McLean, D. Cave, W. Borgen, and P. Slakov, "Coming Home: A Group-Based Approach for Assisting Military Veterans in Transition," *Journal for Specialists in Group Work* 35, 1 (2010): 44–68, https://doi.org/10.1080/01933920903466059.

42 Ibid.

43 L.P. Vromans and R.D. Schweitzer, "Narrative Therapy for Adults with Major Depressive Disorder: Improved Symptom and Interpersonal Outcomes," *Psychotherapy Research* 21, 1 (2011): 4–15, https://doi.org/10.1080/10503301003591792.

44 Ibid.

CONTACT! UNLOAD

Annotated Playscript

GRAHAM W. LEA
with George Belliveau and the Company

Some scenes based on *The Return*
by Linda Hassall (2014)

All productions directed by George Belliveau

Rights to produce, film, or record *Contact!Unload* in whole or in part, in
any medium, or in any language, by any group, amateur or professional, are
retained by the lead author. Interested persons are requested to apply to
graham.lea@umanitoba.ca or george.belliveau@ubc.ca.

Dramatis Personae

Also plays[a]

VET 1
VOICE OF GIRLFRIEND (*Moment 3 & Moment 16*)
WIFE (*Moment 8*)
PARENT (*Moment 8*)
23CHARLIE (*Moment 21*)

VET 2
UNCLE (*Moment 12*)
INFORMANT (*Moment 21*)

VET 3
HOST (*Moment 8*)
FATHER (*Moment 12 & Moment 14*)
APACHE11 (*Moment 21*)

VET 4
DALE
SON (*Moment 8*)
VOICE FROM TABLEAU (*Moment 8*)
PRIEST (*Moment 8*)
BROTHER (*Moment 12*)

TIM
ACTOR
DIRECTOR
COUNSELLOR

---

a   Other casting combinations are possible.

From the Original Program, Spring 2015

Company

Warren Geraghty

Chuck MacKinnon

David Kuhl

Candace Marshall

JS Valdez

Marv Westwood

George Belliveau

Oliver Longman

Tim Garthside

Graham W. Lea

Mike Waterman

Phillip Lopresti

Dale Hamilton

Theatre Production

Producers:
Marv Westwood and George Belliveau

Production Management:
Oliver Longman and JS Valdez

Director:
George Belliveau

Assistant Director:
JS Valdez

Stage Manager:
Graham W. Lea

Musician:
Jon Ochsendorf

Theatre Technician:
Krysten Neeson

Ushers:
Gloria Burke, Maddie Douglas, Sophie Belliveau

Production Assistance:
Anna Keefe

Front of House:
Sara Bynoe

Script by Graham W. Lea and the Man/Art/Action Project Theatre Company, with two scenes adapted from *The Return* by Linda Hassall: Episode 11: "In Service to the Country," and Episode 13: "Living on Edge."

Glossary

RPG: Rocket-propelled grenade

IED: Improvised explosive device

Birds: Helicopters

Zero: Radio call sign for headquarters

Medevac: Medical evacuation

Nine-liner: Communications report used when requesting medevac

Apache11: Radio call sign for Apache attack helicopter. Pronounced "Apache one one"

Contact: Communication report identifying enemy attack

23Charlie: Radio call sign identifying infantry unit. Pronounced "two three Charlie"

Para/Paraprofessional: A graduate of the Veterans Transition Program who assists the leading team

Unfuck your shit: The therapeutic process of working through personal trauma and/or dropping the baggage (Veteran Transition Program slang)

VTN: Veterans Transition Network

Director and Playwright's Note

The development of *Contact!Unload* was a highly collaborative process. The voices of the four veterans offered authenticity and rich content to the piece. Their stories were brought to life in a play-building process that led to this workshop production. Working with this team of veterans and civilians has been a rich and ongoing learning journey. A cornerstone of *Contact!Unload* is the long-standing work of the Veterans Transition Program, and our goal was to honour this work and the stories of our four veterans and all of those who have struggled to return in as truthful a manner as possible.

– George Belliveau, Graham W. Lea, JS Valdez

A Note about the Tribute Pole Artists

With the artistic direction of Foster Eastman and carving lessons by Squamish master carver Xwalacktun, veterans created a tribute pole telling stories of their experiences in Afghanistan. The purpose of this project was to explore alternative methods and meta-cultural experiences to help with the healing process, and to share the veterans' stories in a creative and healing environment.

Carvers

Dale Hamilton	Sean Loucks	Jason Villeneuve	Foster Eastman
Tim Laidler	Jared Reynolds	Bob Sutherland	Ian Morrison

◇◇◇◇◇◇◇◇◇◇

Special Thanks
For help with this workshop production and the Man/Art/Action Project:

Michael Balfour

Linda Hassall

Tim Laidler

Carson Kivari

Ken Lieuwen

Glenn Chatten

Neil Ryan

Blair McLean,
Videographer

Karim Mawani,
Assistant
Videographer

Ernesto Peña,
Graphic Design

Nathan Tessier, Carpenter

Miles Lavkulich and staff
at Studio 1398

Xwalacktun for carving
lessons and cultural guidance

Don Graham for his talents,
generosity, and expertise

Spencer Graham for sound-
track development

Ian Morrison for his skills
and commitment

Candace Marshall for hands-on
carving and caring

Tracy Averill for continual
back-up support

Galen Lofsted for his creative
video vision

Scott Bolton for continual
contributions to veterans'
projects

Renée Sarich for project
management

Take Five Café on Nicola Street
for discounting our regular
coffee/tea

In Canada today, many of us are unaware of the complexities and consequences of war for modern-day veterans in transition. Contact!Unload provides a unique window into the lived experiences of four veterans who perform their own stories of war and transition. Each scene reflects the post-deployment truths and challenges of many returning men and women and their families. The production also showcases Vancouver civilians, artists, and therapists performing alongside veterans. Audience discussion with veterans will follow.

If you know a veteran struggling to transition back after service, find out more at vtncanada.org.

Original Company, Spring 2015

George Belliveau
Tim Garthside
Dale Hamilton
Warren Geraghty
David Kuhl
Graham W. Lea
Oliver Longman
Phillip Lopresti
Chuck MacKinnon
Candace Marshall
JS Valdez

Mike Waterman
Marv Westwood

George Belliveau, Director
JS Valdez, Assistant Director
Graham W. Lea, Lead Writer,
   Stage Manager, Light and Sound
   Designer
Jon Ochsendorf, Musician
Anna Keefe, Production
   Assistance

Touring Company, Fall 2015

George Belliveau
Luke Bokenfohr
Stephen Clews
Warren Geraghty
Chuck MacKinnon
Mike Waterman

George Belliveau, Director
Graham W. Lea, Stage Manager
Phillip Lopresti, Touring Stage
   Manager

Touring Company, Fall 2016

George Belliveau
Luke Bokenfohr
Stephen Clews
Tim Garthside
Tim Laidler
Phillip Lopresti
Chuck MacKinnon

George Belliveau, Director
Eric Double, Dramaturg
Jon Ochsendorf, Musician

Touring Company, Fall 2017

George Belliveau
Luke Bokenfohr
Stephen Clews
Tim Garthside
Tim Laidler
Phillip Lopresti
Chuck MacKinnon
Christopher Gaze[a]

George Belliveau, Director
David Geary, Dramaturg and
   Assistant Director
Graham W. Lea, Stage Manager
Liam Peel, Production Assistant
Carson Kivari, Bernadette Mah,[a]
   and Geoff Gillard,[a] Musicians

---

a   Vancouver performances only.

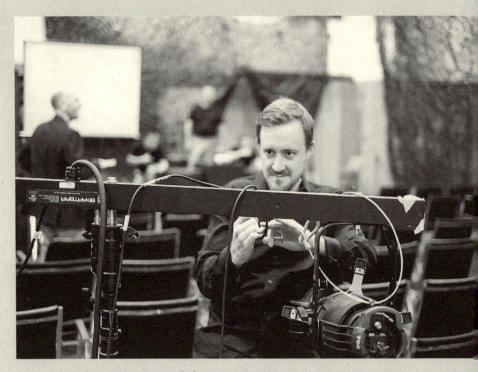

Figure 12 Graham Lea setting up lights | Photo by Blair McLean; used with permission.

SET: *A blank stage. There may be a projection screen stage left (SL) to balance the TRIBUTE POLE.[a] There are four black boxes onstage that serve a variety of purposes throughout the performance.*

COSTUME: *Casual clothing.*

LIGHTING: *A general wash for Shakespeare and therapeutic enactment scenes. A slightly distinguished wash for soldiers' stories, a special on the TRIBUTE POLE, a down centre stage (DCS)[b] special, and possibly down stage right (DSR) and down stage left (DSL) specials. There may also be a special for a musician. TRIBUTE POLE should be as inconspicuous as possible when not illuminated.*

Note: *Transitions between moments should be smooth, with no breaks.*

As the audience enters:
Stage is in dim general lighting with the TRIBUTE POLE special.
Preshow music playing.

If there are any opening speeches, fade the house lights and preshow music before. If not, house lights fade as preshow music segues into the song Black Sedan *by Jon Ochsendorf, which is played live.[c]*

General lighting fades, leaving musician and TRIBUTE POLE specials.

After the song, fade musician special, leaving just the special on the POLE.

Video introducing the TRIBUTE POLE.[d]

---

a See Chapter 6.
b Stage directions are made from the perspective of the actor. Therefore, stage left would refers to the area on the audience's right. Down stage refers to being close to the audience, while upstage is away from the audience.
c "Black Sedan," YouTube video, posted by Rick Colhoun, November 1, 2014, http://www.youtube.com/watch?v=EfHV6ER7PNY.
d "Veterans Tribute Pole Foster Eastman," YouTube video, posted by Foster Eastman, May 5, 2015, http://www.youtube.com/watch?v=5Ol8N9kUfgg.

TRIBUTE POLE raising ceremony. During the ceremony, members of the company and invited guests raise the TRIBUTE POLE.[a]

The song Waiting in Line *by Neil Ryan plays and projections appear on the screen:*[b]

Almost 600,000 veterans in Canada have served since the Korean War.
25% report a difficult return to civilian life.[c]
When they return their scars are not just physical.
These are not numbers, these are people.

As the projections end, actors enter and form a line onstage. The last projection and music fade out. The TRIBUTE POLE is displayed in silence before lights fade out.

---

a   This ceremony honours the members of the Canadian Forces who died in service in Afghanistan, and establishes the pole as the weight holding down TIM.
b   During some productions, the content of the slides was spoken by the actors.
c   Statistics from M.B. MacLean, L. Van Til, J.M. Thompson, J. Sweet, et al., "Postmilitary Adjustment to Civilian Life: Potential Risks and Protective Factors," *Physical Therapy* 94, 8 (2014): 1185–95, https://doi.org/10.2522/ptj.20120107.

◇◇◇◇◇◇◇◇◇◇◇◇◇◇◇◇◇◇

Moment 1: The Line

LOUD MALE VOICE

ATTENTION! *(Lights snap up)* QUICK MARCH! Left, Right, Left ...

ACTORS

(Continuing) Left, Right, Left, Right *(Repeat sotto voce)*

(ACTORS enter quickly and form a line at the lip of the stage. TIM is DSL)

LOUD MALE VOICE

HALT!

◇◇◇◇◇◇◇◇◇◇◇◇◇◇◇◇◇◇◇◇◇◇

Moment 2: Off the Line

ACTOR

(Offstage. At the end of each line there is a gunfire/explosion SFX [sound effect]. With each sound, one person leaves the stage. DALE is the last to leave. At the end, TIM is alone onstage)

What's he that wishes so?[a]
My cousin Westmoreland? No, my fair cousin:
If we are mark'd to die, we are enow
To do our country loss; and if to live,
The fewer men, the greater share of honour.
God's will! I pray thee, wish not one man more.

(TIM crosses US to sit under the TRIBUTE POLE. There is no gunfire as he leaves the line. He puts on headphones around his neck.[b] Lights cross-fade from general wash to isolate TIM alone under the TRIBUTE POLE)

---

a Text from Shakespeare's *Henry V* is adapted from the St. Crispin's Day speech. W. Shakespeare, *The Life of King Henry the Fifth* (1600; repr., Cambridge, MA: The Tech, 1993), IV.iii.21–69, http://shakespeare.mit.edu/henryv/full.html.

b The headphones here and throughout the script were cut in the rehearsal process but are kept in the script as a powerful symbol.

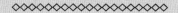

Moment 3: Reach Out #1[a]

VOICE OF GIRLFRIEND

(*Offstage left*)[b] Hey Hon, you wanna go for a movie? You've been down there all day. (*TIM puts headphones on. This is his reaction when people try to talk or reach out to him*)

TIM

Fuck off! (*Remaining light snaps out*)

---

a   Due to casting requirements in touring productions, the girlfriend was replaced with one of the fellow veterans. For the alternate version, see Moment 3 (Alternate) in the Appendix.
b   Having the voice come from offstage left creates a distance between the girlfriend and TIM, who is under the Tribute Pole on stage right. He finally makes the cross to stage left at the end of the performance.

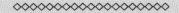

Moment 4: Introduction to Shakespeare

ACTOR

(Lights fade up during the speech. ACTOR enters; he might stand on a box)

> We would not die in that man's company
> That fears his fellowship to die with us.
> This day is called the feast of Crispian:
> He that outlives this day, and comes safe home,
> Will stand a tip-toe when this day is named,
> And rouse him at the name of Crispian.
> He that shall live this day, and see old age,
> Will yearly on the vigil feast his neighbours,
> And say "To-morrow is Saint Crispian:"
> Then will he strip his sleeve and show his scars,
> And say "These wounds I had on Crispian's day."

DIRECTOR

> Okay, great try, but it's not working. It's sounding too much like Branagh, it's too bombastic … there's too much ACTING. *(DIRECTOR gesticulates to try to get the idea across)*

ACTOR

> But it's Shakespeare. It needs to be big. It has that momentum.

DIRECTOR

> I want a different Henry the Fifth. I want to move away from the Olivier grandeur, be more human. St. Crispian was the saint of cobblers, curriers, and tanners. Working men, not soldiers, like these men around you. They've seen battle before. They know they are outnumbered by the French. Convince them to go back, not with music, pomp, and thunder, but with truth, and honesty.

ACTOR

> Truth and honesty? That's not in the script.

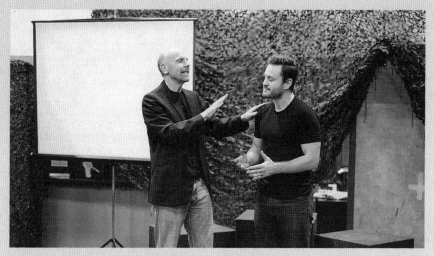

Figure 13 "There's too much ACTING." Left to right: George Belliveau and Mike Waterman | Photo by Blair McLean; used with permission.

DIRECTOR

And to help you get there, I have some guests. Remember those gentlemen we met after rehearsal last week?

ACTOR

I do! They wanted in here when you made us run late.

DIRECTOR

The same. Come on in, gentlemen. *(CHUCK, WARREN, DALE, and COUNSELLOR enter)* Let me introduce [use veterans' names except for TIM], and – *(TIM, sitting under the TRIBUTE POLE, waves that he's not interested).* They're soldiers who have returned from deployment. They work in this space to help make the transition to civilian life.

COUNSELLOR

I work with groups of soldiers like these guys to help them drop their baggage, to unload. Not by sitting around and talking but by acting out and revisiting hard memories, the things they bring back with them. We use enactment to re-create scenes and moments from their past.

ACTOR

Oh, like re-enactment, like reality TV.

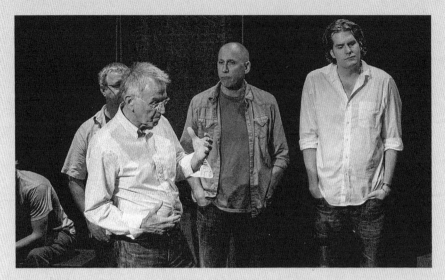

Figure 14 Marv Westwood as COUNSELLOR introduces the veterans. Left to right: Tim Garthside (sitting), Chuck MacKinnon, Marv Westwood, Warren Geraghty, and Dale Hamilton | Photo by Blair McLean; used with permission.

VETs
  NO!

COUNSELLOR
  For some it might be saying goodbye to a friend or sorry to a buddy.

DIRECTOR
  And this is [use counsellor's name], who developed the Veterans Transition Program. They have all agreed to help you work on your speech. Make it more ... real. These men, like the ones you are asking to go into battle, know all too well what it's like to come back. I want you to play off them.

ACTOR
  So, try to convince these guys to go into battle.

DIRECTOR
  Yeah, and I have asked them to stop you anytime a memory is triggered and share their reactions so you know. Help you understand what you are asking your men to do. Got it?

ACTOR

I think so.

DIRECTOR

Capiche?

ACTOR

Capiche.

DIRECTOR

Very good. So, from the top. When you're ready. ACTORS.

ACTOR

What's he that wishes so?
My cousin Westmoreland? No, my fair cousin:
If we are mark'd to die, we are enow
To do our country loss; and if to live –

◇◇◇◇◇◇◇◇◇◇◇◇◇◇◇

Moment 5: It's Fuckin' Awesome

VET 1

(Cuts ACTOR off, highly energized. ACTOR and DIRECTOR do not exit) It's fucking awesome, a fuckin' rush, being mark'd to die, being shot at. I mean it's fucking awesome. I know it sounds strange but it was fucking awesome. You gotta die when you join, so you don't fear dying when you're there. I miss it. Sounds strange ... but I miss it ...

VETs

I miss it.

(VETs form a line of boxes across the stage, slightly on SR. Lighting change. They freeze in tableau. VETs are crouched behind the boxes with guns – anxious but at ease, VET 1 is standing behind them, calm. Live music covers the transition)

VET 2

There'd be days of boredom. Weeks of boredom.

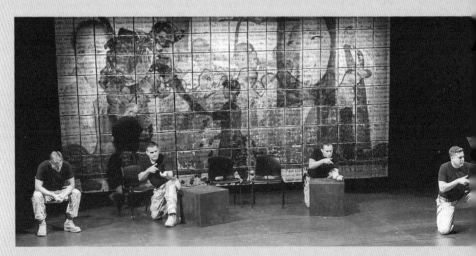

Figure 15 "There'd be days of boredom." Left to right: Tim Garthside, Luke Bokenfohr, Stephen Clews, and Tim Laidler | Photo by the Peter Wall Institute for Advanced Studies; used with permission.

VET 3

Starin' out at a desert that never fucking changes.

VET 2

I've watched that same rock for days.

VET 3

You wait. Wait for those seconds, minutes, those moments.

VET 2

That's what you wait for.

VET 3

Not your family ... over here they can't exist ...

VET 2

They can't exist or you die.

VET 3

So, you wait to get shot. Wait to see if you're going to –

VET 1

Contact! Engage, engage, engage!

(Gunfire, movement, and chaos. Soldiers are shooting toward DSR. Discordant music plays. While it is chaotic, there is order and precision to it, they are doing their job)

Reorg! Reorg! Reorg!

(Actors stand down, reorganize ammunition; VET 1 takes a smoke. They form a tableau) K boys, take a knee. Check yourselves out, make sure you're good to go.

VET 3

How many mags[a] you got?

VET 2

Three. You?

VET 3

Same.

---

a Term used by the Canadian Forces for an ammunition magazine.

VET 2

Fuck, d'you even see what we were shooting?

VET 3

Not a fucking clue man.

VET 2

All I saw was dust.

VET 1

Yeah, that's all your fucking girlfriend sees is dust too.

(Long silence)

VET 3

(To self) Silence.

VET 2

The birds aren't chirping any more.

VET 3

(To self) It's the silence.

VET 2

(To self) Before it begins.

VET 3

(To self) That's what's fucking scary.

VET 2

(To self) You got time to think in the silence.

VET 4

(VET 4 takes a step forward. Those behind him slowly form a tableau of firing rifles) I wanted to be useful. By 2007 it was roadside bombs and suicide bombers. I was standing at the front gate of Kandahar Airfield. This kid, dressed all in black, came right past our red light and big red stop sign. Straight at us. My sergeant is screaming and yelling. I'm thinking, "I'm supposed to do a warning shot first," but the kid is getting closer.

VET 2

60 feet.

VET 3

55 feet.

VET 1

50 feet.

VET 4

There are no barriers between us. He's just a kid. I start to pull the trigger ... hesitate for a split second ... the kid turns his bicycle ... and that was it. I thought, "Shit, maybe that was my one chance to have shot my rifle this entire tour." You know, thank God I didn't, but it's hard to get over wishing you'd done your piece. *(VETs return to the tableau in silence)*

VET 3

Too much time to think in the silence.

(Uncomfortably long silence)

VET 3

(Breathes out) ... fuck

(Long silence, tension)

VET 1

Contact! Engage, engage, engage. Fire, fire, fire.

(Movement and yelling. VET 1 steps out on the boxes as the yelling progresses)

Fucking awesome. The adrenaline kicks in. No time to think. No time to be terrified.

(VETs 2, 3, and 4 stop yelling and exit quickly)

Fucking awesome! I mean, the adrenaline's just pumping. I know I keep saying that. But it's just fucking awesome.

(VET 1 looks around; there is nothing there)

Nothing like it here.
I miss it.
(Breath)
Christ, I miss it.

VETs

I miss it.

DIRECTOR

(To ACTOR in awe) That was ...

ACTOR

...

◇◇◇◇◇◇◇◇◇◇◇◇◇◇◇◇

Moment 6: Reach Out #2

(Lights crossfade to TIM sitting with his headphones on. The theme from
Storage Wars plays. VET 1 enters toward the pool of light, stops, looks at
TIM and then enters)

VET 1

Hey.

TIM

(Distant) hey *(TIM clicks off the TV)*

VET 1

Whatcha doin'?

TIM

nothin'

VET 1

Pretty quiet over here, isn't it?

TIM

yeah

VET 1

You, ahh ... You see the game last night?

TIM

yeah, fucking bullshit

(They sit in a long silence, watching TV. Then VET 1 takes out a cigarette,
hands it to TIM. TIM waves it off and turns slightly away)

VET 1

(Dejected, stands)
Maybe we should do something sometime. You up for that?

TIM

(Hollow) sure

(VET 1 puts hand on TIM's shoulder then exits)

Moment 7: Returning to Shakespeare

DIRECTOR

So you think you can work that rush in? Knowing that some might want to go back. Experience that adrenaline again?

ACTOR

Hard to imagine going back to that but I'll give it a shot. Where from?

DIRECTOR

Let's go from "Then will he roll his cuff."

ACTOR

You mean "strip his sleeve"?

DIRECTOR

Strip his sleeve.

ACTOR

Then will he strip his sleeve and show his scars,
And say "These wounds I had on Crispin's day."
Old men forget: yet all shall be forgot,
But he'll remember with advantages,
What feats he did that day. Then shall our names,
Familiar in his mouth as household words
Be in their flowing cups freshly remember'd.
And Crispin Crispian shall ne'er go by,
From this day to the ending of the world –,

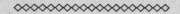

Moment 8: It Shoulda Been Me

VET 2

(*Cutting off ACTOR*) "Freshly remembered." Sure, they'll be remembered in flowing cups ... but not like that, not for feats or fucking celebration.

(*Musician plays "Auld Lang Syne." HOST, WIFE,[a] and SON enter, creating a New Year's Eve party*)

HOST

Hey, guys, welcome, come on in. Good to have you here.

VET 2

How's it goin', man? Hey, who cut your hair, buddy? It's touching your ears again, ya fuckin' hippy!

HOST

(*Hugs wife*) How did someone as beautiful as you end up with him?

WIFE

You missed your chance! Happy New Year.

HOST

So, can I grab you a drink? (*As his back is turned, WIFE glances at VET 2*)

VET 2

What the fuck, what's one more?

WIFE

Thanks.

SON

I'll get it. (*Exits*)

---

a During touring productions, this scene was modified as there were no female company members to play the wife.

P26

HOST

Well, it's great to have you back, man. Happy New Year. Here's to having us all back.

VET 2

(Music stops) Happy New Year?! Happy fucking New Year? What the fuck is wrong with you! *(In his own world)* It shouldn'ta fucking been him. It shoulda been me.

WIFE

I'm sorry, he died ... his friend died this time last year.

VET 2

He was my fucking responsibility. It shoulda been me.

WIFE

An IED.[a] He tried to save him.

VET 2

It shoulda been me ...

WIFE

He was supposed to be in that vehicle.

VET 2

It was my responsibility.

WIFE

They switched places. Last second –

VET 2

Ka-fucking-bang!

(VET 2 and VET 4 form the Survivors' Guilt tableau of an explosion,[b] with VET 2 holding VET 4. VET 1 and VET 3 close in on the tableau with each line. This should all happen very quickly, with overlapping lines)

---

a Improvised explosive device.
b See Figure 21 in Chapter 13.

VET 3[a]

Get out of the vehicle –

VET 1

Try to save his ass –

VET 3

Can't even get the fucking buckle off –

VET 1

Had to cut him out –

VET 3

There was blood everywhere and
sweating –

VET 1

Putting quick clot on him –

VET 3

Burns your hands.

                                        VET 2

                                        It's horrible.

VET 3

Helicopter flying around somewhere
with some goddammed general –

VET 1

I hope he liked his fucking flight –

VET 3

Should be my friend on that
helicopter.

                                        VET 2

                                        It shoulda been me. Come on,
                                        breathe, motherfucker.

                                        VOICE FROM TABLEAU
                                        Mom ... Mom?

---

a   This was originally a long monologue that was later broken up to ease the emotional burden on
    the actor. It also added more dynamism to the scene.

VET 2

Nothin' I could do.

VET 3

Nothin' I could do. Put his head
down ...

VET 1

My hand right there ...
*(Moves the tableau to put VET 3's
hand on the ribcage of VET 1)*

VET 2

I could feel his breath.

VET 3

I could feel his breath.

VET 1

In and out ...

VET 3

Gettin' shallow ...

VET 1

In and out ...

VET 3

Tried to tell him.

VET 2

I ... I ...

VET 1

In and out ...

VET 3

Tried to tell him.

VET 2

(Beat)
It shoulda been me.

VETs 1–3

It shoulda been me.

VET 1

(VETs 1 and 3 enter the scene and pick VET 4 up)
Chopper finally comes –

VET 3

Put him on a stretcher and load him in –

VET 1

Stretcher wouldn't fit in the goddam fucking helicopter –

VET 3

Couldn't close the fucking door –

VET 1

Had to tip him out inside the –

VET 3

Fucking blood everywhere.
(VETs 1, 3, and 4 exit or freeze)

                                        VET 2

                                        (Silence) Last thing I saw was the
                                        soles of his boots.
                                        (Moves to centre) They asked me
                                        to be his Escort Officer. *(Pace
                                        quickens again)*

VET 1

(VETs 1, 3, and 4 enter and form a line slightly behind VET 2)
Shoved into the back of a C-130[a] for 16 hours with the casket.

VET 2

But it shoulda been me.
I asked if I could hang his uniform up somewhere. He wouldn't want to
put it in the overhead compartment. He would want it hung. My friend
was only gonna wear it one last time.

VET 3

Son, do you know where you are?

---

a   C-130 Hercules aircraft.

VET 2

I'm in Canada, I think.

VET 4

Watched them take his casket off the plane. *(All VETs are now in a line and they watch the casket move across the stage)*

VET 1

(One by one, VETs raise their hands)
His five-year-old son put his hand on his dad's casket ...

VET 2

It shoulda been me.

VET 3

No time to grieve.

VET 4

A job to do.

VET 1

We FFFLLLLEEWW down the Highway of Heroes.[a]

VET 2

It was completely empty.

VET 3

On the side of the road firefighters in full uniform –

VET 1

Lights all going –

VET 2

Police saluting –

VET 3

And the people –

---

a When fallen soldiers were repatriated to Canada, they were often taken by convoy along Ontario Highway 401 from Canadian Forces Base Trenton to the coroner in Toronto. Crowds would gather along the route to pay respects. In 2007, this stretch of the 401 was named the Highway of Heroes.

VET 4

Everywhere.

VET 2

Crying for someone they never met, never knew.

VET 1

No time to grieve –

VET 3

A job to do –

VET 2

Support the family. *(Line tableau breaks)*

PRIEST

Ashes to ashes. Dust to dust.

PARENT

(To VET) Thank you for helping my son. He spoke of you often. *(Reluctantly offers him a meticulously folded hockey jersey. VET 2 gently takes the jersey)* It was his favourite. He would have wanted you to have it.

VET 2

A grieving parent's last wish. What the hell am I supposed to do with a used hockey jersey? A Toronto Maple Leafs one at that. *(A sad laugh/ smile)* Fuck.

◇◇◇◇◇◇◇◇◇◇◇◇◇◇◇◇◇◇◇◇

Moment 9: Music #1

(Live musician plays)

(In later productions all VETs would fall asleep on the stage. Sudden gunshot SFX. All VETs wake up as if from a bad dream)

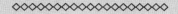

Moment 10: Logic and Chaos

(A tableau is formed. A line of people, back to back. VET 4 begins this abstract movement piece by moving through the line of people. Music continues. TIM is sitting writing in a journal)

TIM[a]
Brilliant and Foolish.
You spend so much time in your own head.

TIM and VET 4
Dualism's the curse of it.

VET 4
Chaos asserts control.
Logic sits back, calculates odds,
only to conclude it's not worth the effort.

When the fuck did it come to this?
When Logic decided that he couldn't deal?
When the both of you saw men, friends, get torn apart for no reason other than luck.
Was that when Logic decided to fold up shop
Let Chaos take the reins?
Saw that Chaos had it right.

But with Chaos in charge, things ain't so fucking good.
I would hate for anyone I love to have a look inside my head.
The yard is overgrown.
No one's paid the bills in months.

A little white pill
A little white pill keeps Chaos on his heels
Ties one hand behind his back

---

a This poem was adapted from some of Dale Hamilton's writing. The poems here and in Moment 13 provide a break from the realistic intensity of the rest of the show. They were cut in later productions.

Brings Logic back to the table to maybe think 'bout being in charge again.

But by the looks of the place ...

VET 4 and TIM
Logic might decide it's not worth the effort.

DIRECTOR
Now that was something.

ACTOR
Would you like –

DIRECTOR
Ssshhh!

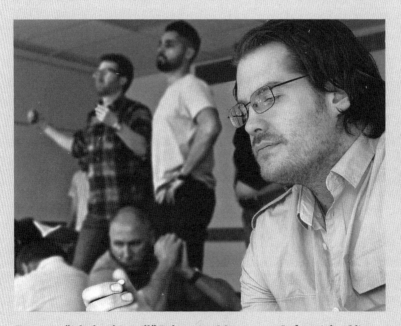

Figure 16 "A little white pill." Rehearsing Moment 10. Left to right: Oliver Longman, Warren Geraghty, Phillip Lopresti, and Dale Hamilton | Photo by Karen Forsyth; used with permission.

◇◇◇◇◇◇◇◇◇◇◇◇◇◇◇◇◇◇

Moment 11: Reach Out #3

(Lights up on TIM in the TRIBUTE POLE special. He is staring off into space. VET 2 enters the stage, comes to the edge of the special)

VET 2

Tim?

TIM

yeah

VET 2

Tim, looks like you're not doin' so well.

TIM

nah, I'm fine

VET 2

Look, Tim. We know it's hard. We've seen fucked up shit too. There's this doctor I see. Helps me a bit.

TIM

I'm fucked up, but not fucked up like you

VET 2

Dude, injury is injury.

TIM

there are guys much worse than me ... I don't need that shit
(Puts on headphones)

VET 2

Tim ...
(TIM turns away. To ACTOR and DIRECTOR) He's not ready.

◇◇◇◇◇◇◇◇◇◇◇◇◇◇◇◇◇◇

Moment 12: Bring It Back and Pass It Around[a]

DIRECTOR

Now, that was something.

ACTOR

I had no idea what they bring back.

VET 4

Most don't. Shit, we often don't know ourselves.

VET 3

We go through hell then bring it back and pass it around.

(They begin to move into a poker scene)

ACTOR

What do you mean?

VET 1

It's not just us that suffer.

VET 2

It's everyone around us.

VET 4

Our friends, families, everyone.

(Improvised poker banter)

BROTHER[b]

K, dad, uncle-big-stacks over there, chips in. *(They do and BROTHER deals)* Deuce of spades, six spades, four spades. Three spades on the table.

---

a In the original production, this was a family scene with mother, father, and son. With no female cast members in the touring version, this was turned into a poker game with an uncle.

b Here, using BROTHER (VET 4), FATHER (VET 3), and UNCLE (VET 2) indicates a shift from speaking to the ACTOR and DIRECTOR to being in the remembered scene.

FATHER

Twenty. *(Chips in)*

UNCLE

Call. *(Chips in, as does BROTHER)*

BROTHER

And a three of spades.

FATHER

Hundred. *(Chips in)*

UNCLE

You're not bluffing your way out this time. *(Chips in)*

FATHER

Me bluff? Never!!

BROTHER

Yeah, right! I'm in too. *(Chips in)* Annddd on the river ...
king of spades.

UNCLE

Jesus, last time I saw a suited flop was when your boy cleaned house!

FATHER

It was the only time he ever cleaned anything!

BROTHER

Yeah, the bastard had a straight flush.

FATHER

Ya know. I was so proud of him being a soldier, like me. Really proud.
Never told him that. I, I always expected my boy to come home, but he
just wasn't the same.[a]

UNCLE

(Trying to offer comfort) It's hard.

---

a Despite the excitement of the great poker hand, the father is hijacked. Through this scene, we
   see various forms of the impact of secondary traumatic stress. See R. Dekel and C.M. Monson,
   "Military-Related Post-Traumatic Stress Disorder and Family Relations: Current Knowledge and
   Future Directions," *Aggression and Violent Behavior* 15, 4 (2010): 303–9, https://doi.org/10.1016/j.
   avb.2010.03.001.

FATHER

He called one day. I could tell something was wrong. I told him to man up, get a coffee, go for a run. He was reaching out and all I could do was tell him to go for a goddamn run. It was just after that he –

UNCLE

No! No, he died as a result of combat.

BROTHER

What are you talking about? He didn't die in Afghanistan, he blew his fuckin' brains out right there in the kitchen.

FATHER

I thought it was a car backfiring.

BROTHER

Dad, he fucking killed –

UNCLE

No, he –

FATHER

NO! He didn't kill himself. His wounds killed him.[a]

UNCLE

Wounds he sustained in a combat zone.

FATHER

It's just as terrible as dying from a bomb or a bullet. No, it's crueler. Takes longer to kill.

BROTHER

It's more vicious. Gets inside ya. Gets inside all of us. *(Exits)*

UNCLE

I'm worried about your younger boy.

FATHER

He just can't get himself together.

---

a   Only when he hears his remaining son repeat his thinking can the father see that his veteran son did indeed succumb to wounds he sustained, even if they were not physical.

UNCLE

He shouldn't a seen that.

FATHER

He's got a camping trip this weekend with the boys. They'll help pull him through.[a]

---

a Here we see the father's care for, but inability to emotionally support, his remaining son. The camping trip with the boys refers to an incident described in A. Ligaya, "Brother of Dead Soldier Missing in BC Interior," *Globe and Mail*, July 24, 2007, http://www.theglobeandmail.com/news/national/brother-of-dead-soldier-missing-in-bc-interior/article689810/.

◇◇◇◇◇◇◇◇◇◇◇◇◇◇◇◇◇◇

Moment 13: Invisible

*(Return to TIM in the TRIBUTE POLE special. TIM reads from his journal.
READER reads from an identical one. The others move chaotically
around TIM, reflecting the text)*

TIM[a]

My thoughts intrude   My thoughts they intrude, resurgent
   Vigilance   With vigilance I seek the insurgents
   Insurgents   Necessary to keep my brothers alive
                                         In this task, together we all strive

TIM and READER

I am helpless when my mind goes   I am helpless when my mind goes
   back   back

READER

Its frequency I've totally lost track   Its frequency I have totally lost track
On the bus, on the train, in the   On the bus, on the train, in the
   street   street
The proof's my hammering heart   The proof, my hammering heart
   beat   beat

Shoulders back, stand tall, be   Shoulders back, stand tall and be
   proud.   proud
How can I?   How can I, when I can't even stand
I can't even stand in a crowd.   in a crowd
Mind races, fists clench, I break   My mind races, fists clench and I
                                          break
Consumed with   Consumed with rage, my sanity at
                                          stake

---

a   This is taken from a poem written by Tim Garthside. It was adapted to lift it off the page more
   smoothly. While Tim approved doing so, he preferred his version, which is included here on the
   right. Originally, Tim performed the whole piece. Later, one of the company members read parts
   of the poem, allowing us to see an outer calm amid a chaotic inner world.

TIM
> RAGE.

READER
> My sanity's at stake.

Threat assessment out of control	Threat assessment I can't control, subversive
The task to relax but I'm in a one-man foxhole.	With this task to relax is preclusive
My resolve to fight through is gritty	My resolve to fight through, it is gritty
For fuel, it don't need your pity	For fuel, it does not require your pity
War has scarred my soul	The experience of war has scarred my soul
And every day I pay the toll.	Each day for their presence, I pay the toll
I'd trade it back to be unaware	I'd trade them back post haste, sweet ignorance
of just how much the world doesn't care.	To know not the capacity of this world's sufferance

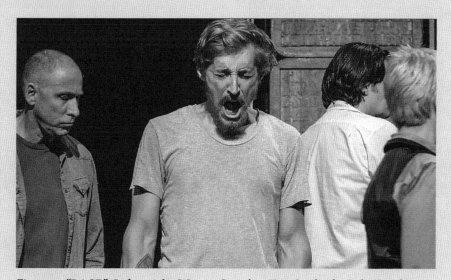

Figure 17 "RAGE." Left to right: Warren Geraghty, Tim Garthside, Dale Hamilton, and Candace Marshall | Photo by Blair McLean; used with permission.

◇◇◇◇◇◇◇◇◇◇◇◇◇◇◇◇◇◇

Moment 14: Reach Out #4

(TIM picks up phone, dials. Phone SFX, FATHER enters with phone)[a]

FATHER

Hello?

TIM

hi dad

FATHER

Tim? It's been a while. How're –

TIM

yeah, yeah it has.

FATHER

What have you been up to?

TIM

you know, nothing much, watchin' TV, staring at the computer

FATHER

Is something wrong? Are you ... something wrong at work?

TIM

No, dad. I'm just ... I'm fine. You wouldn't understand.

FATHER

Well, why don't you get on up, come over for a visit, get a coffee with friends, do something constructive. Go for a run.

TIM

(Dismissive) Yeah, yeah dad, I'll go for a run. *(Tension. TIM hangs up)*

FATHER

A run?! My son. He's reaching out and all I can do is tell him to go for a goddamn run.

---

a FATHER is again played by VET 3

◇◇◇◇◇◇◇◇◇◇◇◇◇◇◇◇◇◇◇◇

Moment 15: Music #2

(Live musician plays)

◇◇◇◇◇◇◇◇◇◇◇◇◇◇◇◇◇◇

Moment 16: Group Reach Out

(Music continues. VETs circle around TIM walking/shopping. They ad lib a wave of voices inviting TIM)

VET 1

Hey, Tim, we haven't seen much of you lately.

VET 2

Let's go out tonight, have a beer.

VET 3

Hang out?

VET 4

Catch the game?

TIM

Would you all just fuck right off!?

(All freeze. Special on TIM)

People all around me. But it's not real. None of it's real. Going fucking shopping. Hundred-dollar shoes, thousand-dollar purses. They don't have a clue. Who cares if your fucking Starbucks coffee's not 180 fucking degrees. FUCK. It's not real. Afghanistan's real. It's something. When I'm there, I'm something. I'm alive. When I'm here, I'm just dead inside.

(Special fades. TIM remains in place. Phone rings)

VOICE OF GIRLFRIEND

(Offstage left) Hey, Hon, let's go out tonight, catch a movie. We haven't gone out all week.

TIM

I told you to fuck off! *(Remaining lights snap out, then return to general wash)*

◇◇◇◇◇◇◇◇◇◇◇◇◇◇◇◇◇◇◇◇◇

Moment 17: Can't Sleep

(Music from Moment 9 returns. All collapse on the floor trying to sleep.
A sudden gunshot SFX wakes them up)

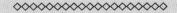

Moment 18: Back to Shakespeare

DIRECTOR

So, what do you think?

ACTOR

I am starting to see more than the romantic "Ra Ra Ra" of war. I've gotta look at things differently. What I need isn't in the script, it's right here.

DIRECTOR

So, you think you can work it in the speech.

ACTOR

I promise to try my best.

DIRECTOR

Very well then. Actors, we'll take it from "then shall our faces."

ACTOR

Names!

DIRECTOR

Right, names.

ACTOR[a]

Then shall our names,
Familiar in his mouth as household words
Be in their flowing cups freshly remember'ed.
And Crispin Crispian shall ne'er go by,
From this day to the ending of the world,
But we in it shall be remember'd;
We few, we happy few, we band of brothers;
For he to-day that sheds his blood with me –

---

a   The ACTOR serves as a proxy for the audience. As he learns these stories and is impacted by them, so too (hopefully) is the audience.

Moment 19: Band of Brothers

DALE

(Musician underscores)
Look, hold on. It's better. But that thing you said, band of brothers. I don't think you know what that really means. Look. This is my band of brothers. *(Points to the bracelet on his wrist, crosses DCS)*[a] It's Nick Bulger, Steven Marshall. It's Andrew Nuttal. It's John Wayne Faught. It's Darren Fitzpatrick, Tyler Todd, Kevin McKay, Byron Greff. Every day. Every fucking day I carry them with me. I left them there. But with my band of brothers I keep them. That is why we went. That is why most of us wanna go back. It's not for you. It's not even for some cause. No cause is enough to keep your body going when it doesn't want to take another step. It's them. It's these guys on my wrist. *(The line from the beginning is formed again. There is a gap where TIM stood at the beginning)* It's the men and women on my left and right. The guys we served with. The ones that came back, the ones that didn't. That is a band of brothers *(Female vet beside DALE elbows him gently)* and sisters. That is why we fought. That's why we keep fighting. And we're still a band. We're still bound.[b]

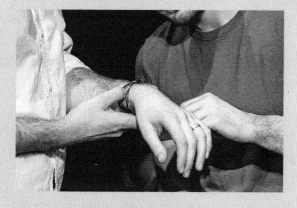

Figure 18 Dale Hamilton showing Mike Waterman his "band of brothers." | Photo by Blair McLean; used with permission.

---

a Dale Hamilton, who played VET 4, wore a bracelet on which were inscribed the names of his friends who died in service in Afghanistan (see Figure 18).
b Through this monologue, DALE comes to the realization that he is bound to fight and has to fight for TIM, and that fighting for him extends beyond the battlefield.

◇◇◇◇◇◇◇◇◇◇◇◇◇◇◇◇◇◇◇

Moment 20: Reach Out #5

DALE

Tim?

TIM

Would you just fuck off!

DALE

Tim, this is fucking enough. You haven't been living for seven years.
I've ... I've been through exactly the same shit. I know what it's about.
But you're turning one casualty into two. You don't have to live like this.
Hope's not at the end of a gun or the bottom of a bottle of pills.

TIM

What choice do I have?

DALE

You've tried this fucking choice. How's it working for you?

TIM

Like fucking shit.

DALE

Yeah, like shit! Look, there's something I did and it helped me. I want
you to come too.

TIM

where

DALE

Does it fucking matter? Not here!

TIM

i don't know man

DALE

Look, in the army they taught us to rely on each other, to trust each
other. You know I have your back, right?

TIM

yeah

DALE

Then just fucking trust me! Look, this is probably going to be the hardest fucking thing you'll ever do. It was for me and it saved my life.

TIM

It saved your life?

DALE

Yeah, it did.

TIM

(Breath) ... okay

DALE

Okay.

(Company enters and walks around creating a cacophony of movement and sound. They all tell their key trauma stories, overlapping each other to establish the therapeutic enactment space. They then stop to greet TIM and welcome him)

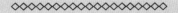

Moment 21: Therapeutic Enactment[a]

COUNSELLOR

Thanks, guys, for welcoming Tim into the group and introducing yourselves. Tim, the way this works is we walk.

TIM

Walk?

COUNSELLOR

And talk. Walk with me. *(COUNSELLOR walks TIM around the stage)* Can you tell us a bit about your story?

TIM

What can I say? I was lucky on my tour. Never shot at, not blown up. The only blood I shed was a goddamn nosebleed 'cause the desert was so fucking dry.

COUNSELLOR

How old were you?

TIM

Twenty-one.

COUNSELLOR

Just twenty-one. That was seven years ago right? *(TIM nods)* You know, Tim, you don't have to be shot at to be not okay.

VET 1

If you go, you've been hurt.

VET 2

We all come back with wounds.

---

a In touring productions, this moment was shortened and reworked to a more storytelling style. See Moment 21 (Alternate) in the Appendix of this playscript. This section was based in large part on an article in *The Tyee* (reprinted in Chapter 4).

COUNSELLOR

These guys, they know.

TIM

(Reluctantly) My trauma happened in an office chair. It sounds fucking stupid. I was traumatized in a fucking office chair. I had my headphones on. *(A veteran brings an office chair or black box. TIM puts headphones on. General wash fades a bit and TIM is shown in a special. COUNSELLOR stays behind TIM)*

It's like you're wearing a trap, this cage on your head all the time. That's where I was on August 3, 2006. Sitting in this fucking office chair.

COUNSELLOR

Tell us what happened.

(SFX: large explosion followed by continued gunfire until stated in the script. The Survivors' Guilt tableau from Moment 8 is recreated SR and may be lit in a blue or green light. ACTOR is seated to the side of the tableau)

23CHARLIE[a]

(From tableau)

Zero,[b] this is 23Charlie – Contact![c] Wait.[d] Out.[e]
23Charlie. Send QRF.[f] We have hit an IED. Taken multiple casualties. Nine-liner[g] to follow. Over.[h]

ACTOR as TIM[i]

Zero. Send. Over.

---

a   It was important to the veterans in the company to be as authentic as possible regarding the language of the field. Pronounced "two three Charlie."

b   This is the radio call name for the signaller. Here, the troop identified as 23CHARLIE is calling from the field to the signaller, TIM.

c   Contact with the enemy.

d   Wait for further information; keep the radio network quiet.

e   Message is complete and others on the radio network can speak.

f   23CHARLIE is requesting the quick reaction force to secure and survey the area.

g   The casualty and evacuation report that consists of nine lines. It includes Who, What, When, Where, Why, and How, then the specifics on the individual casualty (type of injury, triage condition, service number, and nationality).

h   Message is complete but conversation is not.

i   In the first production, the ACTOR portrayed TIM in the field, and Tim portrayed TIM in the therapeutic enactment. It could also be presented with one actor doing both parts.

23CHARLIE

23Charlie. Nine-liner: four without vitals. One zero Priority 1 and 2.[a]
Over.

TIM

Four killed, ten wounded.
It was the wounded.

23CHARLIE

Zero, this is 23Charlie. Send medevac. We need extraction ASAP! Over.

TIM

The wounded.

23CHARLIE

Zero, this is 23Charlie. We are taking effective enemy fire from a
compound southeast of our position. Over.

TIM

(To COUNSELLOR) It's protocol. The medevac birds will not fly if there
is effective enemy fire.

ACTOR as TIM

23Charlie, this is Zero. Negative on extraction. Hold your position until
the incoming fire is suppressed.

TIM

There's no one coming.

23CHARLIE

Zero, this is 23Charlie. These men are dying. We need a medevac NOW!

ACTOR as TIM

Zero. Negative. Hold your position.

TIM

There's no one coming.

ACTOR as TIM

No one's coming.

---

a Ten wounded at two different priority levels.

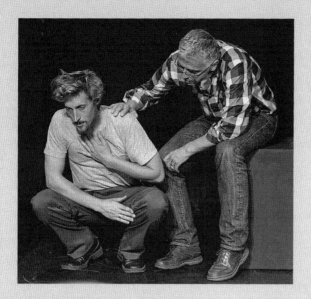

Figure 19 "Tight in the chest." Tim Garthside with Dr. David Kuhl (COUNSELLOR) | Photo by Blair McLean; used with permission.

TIM

No one's coming ... *(COUNSELLOR puts his hand on TIM's shoulder)*

COUNSELLOR

Good, Tim. What's happening in your body?

TIM

Tight in the chest. I'm all hunched over, completely numb.

COUNSELLOR

Okay, Tim, so before you go on, let's get you to take a breath. I'll do it with you. In and out. In and out.[a] When you're ready, go on.

TIM

At the same time, an attack force was on its way, helicopters, bombers, fixed-wing aircraft. They were coming in from everywhere. *(Some actors take places behind TIM)*

APACHE11[b]

(In a calmly authoritative American accent) Zero, this is Apache11. Request coordinates for troops in contact. Over.

---

a This harks back to the Survivors' Guilt scene in Moment 8. It was possible to see audience members breathing with TIM.
b Pronounced "Apache one one."

INFORMANT

Compound at Quebec Alpha 45632 45076.[a]

Red roof with green gate. Everyone inside is Talib.[b]

(INFORMANT continues to repeat coordinates and instructions)

TIM

(To COUNSELLOR) We had an informant on the ground. Giving me the location of the firefight.

ACTOR as TIM

Apache11, this is Zero. Target at Quebec Alpha 45632 45076. Red roof with green gate. Everyone inside is enemy personnel. Eliminate the threat. Over.

APACHE11

Zero, Apache11. On location. *(SFX explosion, gunfire stops)* All enemy targets neutralized. Secondary target on roof holding RPG.[c] Do we engage? Over.

TIM

Roger, Apache11. Neutralize the RPG. Over.

(Silence, then LOUD explosion and bright light, then blackout. In the brightness the INFORMANT and SURVIVORS' GUILT tableau exit)

APACHE11

Zero, Apache11. Enemy target neutralized. We cut him in half. Returning home. Out. *(Exits)*

TIM

(To COUNSELLOR) I ordered him killed. That guy on the roof with the RPG, he was the informant. I killed him. He was trying to help us. He was trying to save the troops bleeding out on the ground. I killed him. This is exactly what I fucking deserve. *(Big pause)*

---

a   Each number is called individually. Some numbers are pronounced differently so they are clearer in transmission and not confused with other numbers. For example, 3 is pronounced as "tree," 5 as "fife," and 9 as "niner."

b   Dari for Taliban.

c   Rocket-propelled grenade.

COUNSELLOR

Tim, if I understand you correctly, you had no idea that the guy on the roof with the RPG was the informant. Right?

TIM

What difference does it make, no, he's still dead.

COUNSELLOR

Just a minute. We're going to do something here. Dale, sit down there, please. *(DALE takes TIM's place)* Look at him, Tim, he's going to be your double, all right? Now imagine he just told you that story. What would you say to him?

TIM

(To DALE, sounding hollow) it's not your fault
(Pause) all I want is for you to feel better

COUNSELLOR

Tim, take off those headphones. *(TIM puts headphones around his neck)* Look at him. Look at yourself. Do you see him? What do you want to say ...?

TIM

(To DALE) it's not your fault

(To COUNSELLOR) But it is. He ordered that guy dead. He killed him.

COUNSELLOR

So it's his fault.

TIM

It's his fault and there's nothing he can do about it.

COUNSELLOR

Look at him. Don't you want him to feel better?

TIM

i need him to feel better

COUNSELLOR

So this person has to suffer the rest of his life for this?

TIM

i don't want ...

COUNSELLOR

No, you don't want him to suffer. Can you forgive him?

TIM

i want to ... But ... *(Pause)*

VET 2 (who played INFORMANT)

I forgive you, Tim. *(Chorus of agreements)*

COUNSELLOR

He wants to be forgiven. What else do you hear?

VET 1

He's stuck.

COUNSELLOR

He's stuck because ...?

VET 4

Because he can't forgive himself yet.

COUNSELLOR

Not yet, but he wants to, doesn't he?

VET 3

He might not be able to, but I forgive him. *(Chorus of agreements)*

COUNSELLOR

So, Tim, you've taken your first step, haven't you? You've looked at yourself. They've looked at you. They've seen you. They forgive you. Even if you can't forgive yourself, yet.

TIM

i need to

COUNSELLOR

You need to because ...

TIM

because if i could forgive him ...

COUNSELLOR

... and forgive myself ...

TIM

and forgive myself ...

COUNSELLOR

Then what?

TIM

Maybe I could ... start to live again.

COUNSELLOR

Out of the dark and into some light. What do you need to keep going?

TIM

More of this

COUNSELLOR

More ...?

TIM

more feeling

COUNSELLOR

And with more feeling ...?

TIM

More life! I haven't been alive for seven years.

COUNSELLOR

That's a long time, seven years. And coming to life is important. That's a big piece of work you've done. These guys have heard you. Take a break and we'll hear from them.

VET 3

I never tire of that lightbulb moment. That's why I keep coming back as a para.[a] To see someone realize they don't have to live with their baggage. I get as much out of that as I did out of my own enactment.

---

a Paras are peers who have been through the therapeutic enactment process and are there to provide support during the enactment.

VET 4

My enactment ... it saved me. I, I was drowning, treading water with a weight around my ankles. Don't get me wrong; it's not all rosy now. But it's a step.

VET 1

It took me nearly twenty years to deal with my shit. I had to do it for me, for my family.

VET IN AUDIENCE[a]

(From audience) You know, I get something out of it every time I see it happening. Being a witness to your enactment is actually helping me.

VET 2

I carried a lot of anger. Everything would be fine, then I'd fucking blow. I'd be hijacked. But these fucking VTN[b] guys, they dragged me through my shit. They helped me unload.

TIM

Ya know, I'm starting to see how much strength it takes to unfuck your shit.

COUNSELLOR

Tim, you've worked hard, dropped some baggage. Feel lighter?

TIM

Yeah. Here with you guys. I don't feel alone any more. You fuckers.

COUNSELLOR

You're not. Let's call it a day, guys. We'll go next door and grab a bite.

(All exit stage left except DALE and TIM. TIM puts headphones on the box. Music underscore starts: Turning Point *by Neil Ryan)*

DALE

Well ...

---

a   When a veteran who had been through the VTP was in the audience, he/she was encouraged to share.

b   Veterans Transition Network.

TIM

That was the hardest fucking thing I've ever had to do. Those sons of bitches made me go back. It fucking sucked.

DALE

Yup, it does. But it's worth it.

TIM

Yeah.

DALE

Coming with us?

TIM

Yeah, I'll catch up. *(DALE exits SL)* I just gotta make a call. *(Takes phone from pocket)* Hey Hon, you wanna catch a movie tonight? *(Beat)* Yeah, I'm ready now. *(TIM exits SL as lights fade, leaving the DCS special on the box with the headphones. Cross-fade to TRIBUTE POLE special MUSIC. All lights are out except the TRIBUTE POLE special)*

Moment 22: Shakespeare Finale

(One by one, the company lines up on the lip of the stage, mirroring the play's first moment)

DIRECTOR
This day is called the feast of Crispian:

ACTOR
He that outlives this day, and comes safe home,
Will stand a tip-toe when this day is named,

VET 1
And rouse him at the name of Crispian.

VET 2
He that shall live this day, and see old age,

VET 3
Will yearly on the vigil feast his neighbours,

VET 4
And say "To-morrow is Saint Crispian:"

TIM
Then will he strip his sleeve and show his scars,

ALL
And say "These wounds I had on Crispian's day."

◇◇◇◇◇◇◇◇◇◇◇◇◇◇◇◇

Moment 23: Finale

(The following text appears as projections on the screen)[a]

> Since 2000 the Veterans Transition Network has helped over 900 veterans transition to civilian life.
> There are many more men and women living in silence.
> If you or anyone you know is in crisis, please talk to one of our onsite counsellors.
> When soldiers return, their scars are not just physical.
> But there is hope.

(Cast forms a line across the stage. They bow, look to the TRIBUTE POLE, bow again. They leave the stage in supportive modes. Lights return to preshow)

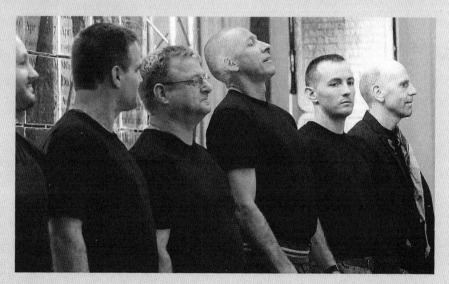

Figure 20 Curtain call at Canada House, November 2015. Left to right: Mike Waterman, Luke Bokenfohr, Chuck MacKinnon, Warren Geraghty, Stephen Clews, and George Belliveau | Photo by Blair McLean; used with permission.

---

a   In the touring productions, these lines were spoken by the veterans.

APPENDIX

◇◇◇◇◇◇◇◇◇◇◇◇◇◇◇◇◇◇◇

Moment 3 (Alternate):
Reach Out #1 (Touring Version)

VET 4

(Crossing to TIM) Hey.

TIM

(Distant) hey

VET 4

Whatcha doin'?

TIM

nothin'

VET 4

Pretty quiet over here, isn't it?

TIM

yeah

VET 4

(Standing, dejected) Maybe we should do something sometime.
You up for that?

TIM

(Hollow) sure ... maybe another time

◇◇◇◇◇◇◇◇◇◇◇◇◇◇◇◇◇◇◇

Moment 21 (Alternate):
Therapeutic Enactment (Touring Version)

COUNSELLOR

Thanks, guys, for welcoming Tim into the group and introducing yourselves. Tim, the way this works is we walk.

TIM

Walk?

COUNSELLOR

And talk. Walk with me *(COUNSELLOR walks TIM around the stage for a while before talking)* Now, can you tell us a bit about your story?

TIM

What can I say? I was lucky on my tour. Never shot at, not blown up. The only blood I shed was a goddamn nosebleed cause the desert was so fucking dry. *(Awkward laugh)*

COUNSELLOR

You know Tim, you don't have to be shot at to be not okay.

VET 1

If you go, you've been hurt.

VET 2

Nobody comes back without wounds.

COUNSELLOR

These guys, they know.

TIM

(Reluctantly) It happened in an office chair. It sounds fucking stupid. I was traumatized in a fucking office chair. I had my headphones on. *(A veteran brings an office chair or black box. COUNSELLOR stays behind TIM)* It's like you're wearing a trap, this cage on your head all the time. That's where I was on August 3, 2006. Sitting in this fucking office chair.

COUNSELLOR

Tell us what happened. *(Discordant music)*

TIM

An IED blew up a convoy. Four killed, ten wounded. It was the wounded. After the explosions the troops began receiving enemy fire from a nearby compound. But there was nothing I could do. It's protocol. The medevac birds will not fly if there is effective enemy fire. These men were dying, painfully ... and I was denying them any hope of survival ... There's no one coming, I told them ... There was no one coming ... They just kept asking.
An attack force – helicopters – flew in from everywhere. An informant on the ground was giving me the location of the firefight. Red roof with green gate. There was a secondary target on the roof holding an RPG ... Do we engage? Do we engage?
Roger. Neutralize the RPG *(Big pause)* They cut him in half.
I ordered him killed. That guy on the roof with the RPG, he was the informant. I killed him. He was trying to help us. He was trying to save the troops bleeding out on the ground. I killed him. This is exactly what I fucking deserve. *(Big pause)*

COUNSELLOR

Tim, if I understand you correctly, you had no idea that the guy on the roof with the RPG was the informant. Isn't that right?

TIM

What difference does it make, no, he's still dead.

COUNSELLOR

Just a minute. We're going to do something here. Stephen, sit down there, please. *(STEPHEN takes TIM's place)* Look at him, Tim, he's going to be your double, all right? Now imagine he just told you that story. What would you say to him?

TIM

(To VET, sounding hollow) it's not your fault. *(Pause)* all i want is for you to feel better

COUNSELLOR

Tim, look at him. Look at yourself. Do you see him? What do you want to say ...?

TIM

(To STEPHEN) it's not your fault. (To COUNSELLOR) But it is. He ordered that guy dead. He killed him.

COUNSELLOR

So, it's his fault.

TIM

It's his fault and there's nothing he can do about it.

COUNSELLOR

Look at him. Don't you want him to feel better?

TIM

i need him to feel better

COUNSELLOR

So this person has to suffer the rest of his life for this? Or, can you forgive him?

TIM

i want to ... but ...

VET 3

We forgive you, Tim. (Chorus of agreements)

COUNSELLOR

So, Tim, you've taken your first step, haven't you? You've looked at yourself. They've seen you. They've forgiven you. Even if you can't forgive yourself (Pause) yet.

TIM

i need to ... because if i could ... forgive him ...

COUNSELLOR

... and forgive myself ...

TIM

and forgive myself ... Maybe I could start to ... to live again.

COUNSELLOR

So, what do you need to keep going?

TIM

More of this. More life! I haven't been alive for ten years.

COUNSELLOR

That's a long time, ten years. Tim, take a break and let's hear from the guys.

VET 1

I never tire of that lightbulb moment. That's why I keep coming back as a para. To see someone realize they don't have to live with that baggage.

VET 2

My enactment ... it saved me. I was drowning, treading water with a weight around my ankles. Don't get me wrong; it's not all rosy now. But it's a step.

VET 3

I carried a lot of anger. Everything would be fine, then I'd fucking blow. I'd be hijacked. But these fucking VTN guys, they dragged me through shit. Helped me unload.

TIM

Ya know, I'm starting to see how much strength it takes to unfuck your shit.

COUNSELLOR

Tim, you've worked hard, dropped some baggage. Feels lighter?

TIM

Yeah. Here with you guys. I don't feel *(Pause)* alone any more. You fuckers!

COUNSELLOR

Let's call it a day, guys. *(All exit stage left except STEPHEN and TIM)*

VET 4

Well ...

TIM

That was the hardest fucking thing I've ever had to do. Those sons of bitches made me go back. It fucking sucked.

VET 4

Yup, it does. But it's worth it.

TIM

Yeah.

Part 2
Performing, Witnessing, and Evaluating

11
Finding My Truth

Timothy Garthside

One does not become enlightened by imagining figures of light, but by making the darkness conscious.

– CARL JUNG[1]

MY GRANDFATHER ONCE told me that when you don't know where you are going in life, any road will get you there. This idiom led me into my adult life, pushed me to volunteer to deploy to Afghanistan on Task Force ORION 01/06 (part of Operation Archer), and, almost ten years later, to seek help for crippling anxiety, insomnia, and major depression. At twenty-one, my interpretation was rather simple: I had no direction in life for my youthful and naïve energies, and deployment to a war zone let me channel that energy into the selfless ideals of military life. My interpretation of this idiom is now rather different and drives me in a very different manner. It has proven to be a powerful force in my life, and I will explain how I came to know this piece of wisdom intimately and the journey on which it has led me.

In the fall of 2012, I had lost my will to continue living. I had tried most everything I could think of to slake this uncomfortable deadness that seemed to have crept into my Soul. I had no idea what post-traumatic stress (PTS) was, or that my experiences in Afghanistan were enough to cause hardship. Through what I now see as much more than luck, in a few weeks I was attending the Veterans Transition Program (VTP) and learning that I had suffered trauma and needed to drop some baggage in order to continue living. Those ten days not only changed my life, honestly, they saved it.

Through a slow process akin to thawing, I began to realize how dead my life had become. Devoid of real personal contact, I had alienated myself from friends and family – I lived, breathed, and bled my employment as a tower crane mechanic. I began to realize that at twenty-nine, I had been running and hiding from my true Self for years, and that back in August of 2006, on the worst day of my life, I shut off my emotions in a bid for self-preservation.

Understanding that as human beings we can make decisions without conscious intention is difficult to grasp, especially when our lives revolve so much around control (e.g., control of behaviour, emotions, life). Life seems much more manageable when we feel we are exercising control over it. The problem I found with this way of life is that we become so busy managing our lives and emotions that we forget to actually live and be present in our everyday. I became so thoroughly lost in trying to control my life that I stopped wanting to live it. This is an extreme reaction but as I have come to understand, it was a normal reaction to abnormal circumstances. Carl Jung once said, "People will do anything, no matter how absurd, in order to avoid facing their own souls."[2]

My first step in understanding myself was learning about authenticity. Authenticity is being true to one's own personality, spirit, or character. It was described to me for the first time as one's inner life being reflected in their outer life, meaning that the way you behave and carry out your life is reflected in how you truly feel inside your own depths. To live authentically does not mean living your life by imbibing every whim and fancy that is tickled; it means knowing oneself and being as true to that as life allows at any given moment. This last piece was essential for my understanding of authenticity. We always strive to live an ideal life and be our ideal selves, but no one ever tells us that because our world isn't *ideal*, it is impossible to live as our ideal selves. The best I can do is to live as a force for good, to be honest and forthright, and do my best to reflect who I feel I am to the world.

To begin living authentically, I had to discover my emotional Self and uncover what my Truth really looks and feels like. The hard and fast way to begin this process is to start looking at your life objectively and reflect on what pleases you and what does not. If those things you found unpleasant could not be rectified, it becomes apparent over much reflection what you can and cannot not live with. This is the foundation of what is true for you, me, and everyone in between. Once we start to uncover our Truth and our sensibilities, it is time to start advocating for what we need in life. My next step was to start speaking my Truth.

Speaking your Truth sounds simple enough and it can be, but it requires intestinal fortitude. In my experience, the times when it has been most difficult to speak my Truth have also proved to be the most important. It is in these moments that authenticity and trusting oneself are the pillars on which we must build our lives. Believing that what matters to you is important enough to take a stand and to fight for is the foundation of the life I am carving out for myself.

In my life, I have had to do things that run completely against the grain of my moral fibre. I believed for many years that this made me a monster and that, should anyone see the things I have hidden deep down inside, they would abhor me. As you may guess, this led to isolation, social anxiety, and a general fear of myself and of what I am capable of. Staring into the abyss of my unlived life was terrifying. There was so much emotion bursting out of the seams that to keep a lid on things I had become so controlled in my bodily movements that I almost resembled an automaton.

Through the VTP and my growing understanding of Self, I began feeling something new. Every time I was faced with a decision, my usual mode of action was to do what I thought I was supposed to do. This means living another's Truth or, worse yet, living what you think others think is the Truth. As it turned out, I had to learn that what is right for one is not necessarily right for all. Once I realized that no one knows my best interests but me, I began to live my Truth. Speaking and living one's own Truth takes strength and faith in one's Self; but fear not, for as I have learned, the vulnerability required is the ultimate display of strength. Only through lifting the armour that we spent our entire lives building can we truly be vulnerable and allow our Truth to shine through. Nothing takes more courage and bravery than baring one's Soul for the world to see. In my experience, this is the only way to let myself be free and unburdened of others' expectations and to live my Truth authentically.

My participation in *Contact!Unload* forced me to take a step out of knowing my Truth and step into fully living it. By performing my trauma in front of hundreds of people, I could no longer hide behind the wall I had built to protect myself.

Those first three performances absolutely drained me, but afterwards I felt different in a new way. I had been freed of my own trappings around my trauma and what others thought of it and of me. I had shed something big, something that had been weighing me down for many years. I no longer carried my story as a burden, a cross to bear, as something that bent and distorted my being. It became an experience that ultimately led to a proverbial rising from the ashes. Only by walking so far down a road to nowhere could I become acutely aware of what it is I want from life. Knowing what you do not want from life can be just as valuable as knowing what it is you do want. I have found the former list much easier to compile and far more meaningful to the individual as it is based purely on one's own experience in life.

I am grateful every single day for the path my life has taken since I decided to continue living. My participation in the VTP and *Contact!Unload* have been instrumental in my path to self-discovery and healing. These two endeavours have also proven to be the hardest, most taxing things I have ever undertaken. Entering back into my own personal hell and fighting my way out to save my Soul has been extremely difficult but necessary. Life without Soul is mere existence. I have found my Truth. I have chosen to thrive.

Notes

1 C.G. Jung, "The Philosophical Tree," trans. R.F.C. Hull, in *The Collected Works of C.G. Jung*, vol. 13, *Alchemical Studies*, ed. G. Alder and R.F.C. Hull (Princeton, NJ: Princeton University Press, 1967; originally published 1945), 265–66.
2 C.G. Jung, "The Symbolism of the Mandala," trans. R.F.C. Hull, in *The Collected Works of C.G. Jung*, vol. 12, *Psychology and Alchemy*, 2nd ed., ed. G. Alder and R.F.C. Hull (Princeton, NJ: Princeton University Press, 1968; originally published 1944), 99–101.

12
Unpacking *Contact!Unload* Using Relational-Cultural Theory

Candace Marshall with Graham W. Lea

Man is a knot into which relationships are tied.

– ANTOINE DE SAINT-EXUPÉRY

MY PARTICIPATION IN *Contact!Unload* began with an invitation from one of my professors, Dr. Marv Westwood. My experience was somewhat unique because of the various roles required of me, including clinical counsellor, research assistant, participant observer, actor, and civilian. Importantly, each of these roles all had something in common: connection to others. My understandings of the project and my roles are situated within the fundamental understanding that human beings are hardwired to be in relationships with others.[1]

For members of the armed forces, the innate need for connection places veterans (especially those affected by post-traumatic stress disorder, or PTSD) at a disadvantage given factors that can potentially keep them isolated from others, including:

- mistrust of anyone outside of the military[2]
- military culture that promotes traditional male socialization and culturally accepted norms of masculinity[3]
- negative effects of PTSD such as hyperarousal, numbing and avoidance, and re-experiencing of traumatic events, and how those symptoms negatively affect the totality of a veteran's lived experience[4]
- men's help-seeking behaviours.[5]

Group approaches are one way to address veterans' experiences of isolation. Vitali Rozynko and Harvey Dondershine argue that homogeneous veteran group interventions are effective at reducing veterans' experiences of isolation through a mutually supportive environment where group members share common experiences and feel safe to express their emotions.[6] Salient to the unpacking of *Contact!Unload* is recognizing that it was not a homogeneous but rather a heterogeneous group. As such, it is important to consider two key naturally occurring social phenomena: 1) ingroups and outgroups (e.g., the veterans and civilians, respectively), and 2) the importance of a common ingroup identity.[7] Michael Hogg suggests that "groups exist by virtue of there being outgroups. For a collection of people to be in a group there must, logically, be other people who are not in the group."[8] Hence, from a social psychology view, the success of *Contact!Unload* hinged on the transformation of the ingroup (veteran)/outgroup (non-veteran) dynamic to a common ingroup identity that would function as one superordinate group.[9] Importantly, Samuel Gaertner and colleagues also note that developing a superordinate group that would blur the boundaries that separated us (veterans) from them (civilians) towards a more inclusive 'we' does not require that a subgroup (e.g., the veterans) abandon its ingroup status or identity.[10]

Perspective Is Everything

In my clinical counselling and psychotherapy practice, I often talk about perspective with clients. Acknowledging one's perspective is important as it forms the basis of our attitudes and shapes our points of view. As a mental health practitioner, my theoretical orientation is rooted in Jean Baker Miller's feminist relational-cultural theory (RCT).[11] As such, I acknowledge that my observations and experiences and the writing that follows are deeply influenced by that perspective.

Relational-Cultural Theory

On the surface, RCT may appear to be an ill-matched framework in which to situate *Contact!Unload,* given feminism's historical focus on women's issues.[12] However, the guiding philosophy of RCT is based on inclusivity.[13] Specifically, RCT recognizes the impact of socio-political and psycho-social factors that influence and shape human development and shape relational patterns with others. According to RCT, healthy relationships are the core of human development and isolation from others is the principal source of human suffering,[14] a claim supported by neurobiology research.[15]

Judith Jordan writes that RCT is rooted in the belief that all "healing" takes place within mutually empathetic, *growth-fostering relationships* that identify and demystify the personal and social factors that become obstacles that prevent mutuality and connectedness to others:[16] "People need to be in connection in order to change, open up, shift, transform, heal, and grow."[17] Hence, a primary goal within RCT is helping people move from isolation to connection through mature growth-fostering relationships that are based on authenticity, honest feedback, and mutual empathy.[18]

According to Jordan, RCT is rooted in three core beliefs.[19] First, the central relational paradox occurs when our innate need to be in connection with others is thwarted by attitudes and behaviours that distance us from the relationships we crave. As a result, we are not genuine within our relationships, concealing our full experience and moving us further into isolation from our relationships with others and ourselves. On the other hand, when we are authentic in our interactions with others, we can move out of isolation and into connection. Second, we form relational images that inform our expectations of future relationships based on our previous relational experiences. Third, each of us has the potential for improving our relational resiliency, the ability to move from disconnection to connection and reconnection with ourselves and others.

Recently, RCT has expanded its focus and addressed factors specific to working with men by acknowledging the gender-specific influences that challenge men's connection and disconnection within their relationships based on the multiple roles in which men operate and the contexts in which they occur.[20] Thelma Duffey and Shane Haberstroh note that men's perspectives of their connections to others is fluid and complex and further complicated by what they describe as self-aggrandizing and self-denigrating perspectives.[21] Self-aggrandizing men dehumanize themselves and others by rejecting personal vulnerabilities while exploiting the same vulnerabilities in others. In essence, vulnerability is interpreted as weakness, whereas control and power over others is seen as a strength. Conversely, when men are self-denigrating, they reject both the value and credibility of their own worth. Hence, RCT recognizes the importance of helping men increase "clarity and balance in their understanding of themselves and others."[22]

In the Beginning: Group Building and Theatre Basics
In group counselling, the most important aspects of the beginning stage of group development are:

- introductions
- discussion of topics
- review of the purpose of the group
- explanation of what to expect from the group
- development of group norms that characterize how the group will operate
- assessment of individual comfort within the group.[23]

Key to this stage of the development of *Contact!Unload* was how Marv Westwood and theatrical lead Dr. George Belliveau would guide group members in creating what therapists often call a "container" that safely holds the group as a whole.[24]

Using a bicycle as a metaphor, Marv was the "hub" from which the spokes of the wheel of *Contact!Unload* would radiate. His status among the veterans was akin to that of an honorary general, given his instrumental role in each of their healing experiences, his dedication and work with fellow veterans, and his role in establishing the Veterans Transition Network (VTN). In addition, Marv's expertise as a master group therapist would guide the pace at which group building between the veterans and civilians would initially develop. George, on the other hand, was the "pedal" and "gear" that transformed the project into motion. With the introduction of theatre exercises, George invited group members to expand their comfort with developing their "performing selves" within the context of performing with "others," and advanced trust and group cohesion through a different kind of risk-taking.

Group Building

Three naturally occurring events characterize the initial group-building stage: 1) the ingroup/outgroup dynamic, 2) the veterans' mistrust of civilians, and 3) the civilians' desire to be accepted by the veterans.

During the first meeting of what would become the company of *Contact!-Unload,* Marv asked the veterans to introduce themselves and share why they had accepted his invitation to be involved. As each of the veterans introduced themselves, they stated in one way or another that their primary motivation was the hope that sharing their experiences might prevent another veteran from taking his or her own life. Additionally, the veterans also expressed:

- curiosity and skepticism about the project
- trepidation about performing
- apprehension about not being heard or understood
- fear that their military service would be criticized
- uncertainty about working with a group of unknown civilians
- uncertainty about whether all of their time, efforts, and sacrifices would be enough to satisfy their motivation and provide them with evidence that they had been able to successfully complete what some of them described in military jargon as "the mission."

One veteran sometimes flexed his ingroup muscle by letting the non-veterans know that, for him, there was a clear distinction between his military mates and his "civi" mates. Adopting a self-aggrandizing stance, he purposely and force-fully bellowed at the civilians, "I know why I'm here, why the FUCK are you here?" This mistrust seemed to convey an embedded belief system that protected his disconnection with others and highlighted the naturally occurring ingroup/outgroup dynamic. Ultimately, the veterans did express a willingness to engage with the civilians, but their trust would have to be earned. Viewed through an RCT lens, shifting relational images and the development of relational resilience that would lead to growth-fostering relationships was still in its infancy.

When the civilians were invited to introduce themselves, there was a communal nervousness. As a group we had unspoken concerns: Would our answers satisfy the veterans' expectations of what was acceptable motivation? Would our motivations be enough to foster a sense of trust and mutual respect? One by one, members of the outgroup carefully introduced themselves and adopted a self-denigrating role that was thrust upon us by the veteran who wielded his power and veteran status. It was made clear in no uncertain terms that we civilians would have to prove our personal worth and trustworthiness. As a group, we quickly recognized that to do this effectively, we needed the veterans' acceptance. Thus, the members of the outgroup were keen to prove their worth and trustworthiness. Almost every person expressed thanks and appreciation for the veterans' service and described both familial military ties as well as personal losses due to suicide. More personally, a few group members also disclosed their own challenges with mental health. Through these self-disclosures, it felt as if outgroup members were attempting to shift long-held relational images that would enable this ingroup of male veterans to better recognize our trustworthiness and personal worth.

Theatre Basics

George's first task was to lead the two groups into the unchartered waters of developing their performing selves. With the introduction of the very first drama exercise, it was apparent that everyone, especially the non-theatre professionals, felt a sense of trepidation, not knowing what was expected or the degree to which each person could meet those expectations. Nonetheless, engaging the veterans and civilians in continued drama exercises over the course of the first month resulted in three major evolutions: 1) increased comfort with performing, 2) increased trust among and between group members, and 3) development of a common group identity.

Utilizing basic physical and vocal theatre exercises, George presented creative opportunities for each individual to become more comfortable with their body and voice. As comfort with the performing self grew, George immersed the group in more challenging exercises that brought us in direct physical contact with one another. These exercises facilitated the development of trusting and supportive relationships that translated into taking bigger personal risks and greater comfort with performing authentically with others.

All together and repeat after me: "A big black bug bit a big black bear, made the big black bear bleed blood" (warm-up exercise).

From their initial introduction, these exercises became a part of every rehearsal and were vital in creating common experiences.[25] With time, these exercises no longer aroused suspicion but became something the entire company looked forward to and actively engaged in with increasing levels of personal commitment, intensity, and creativity. As a result, trust began to deepen among group members as they engaged authentically and compassionately with one another – testimony that as a group, we were moving out of isolation and disconnection into connection by way of shifting relational images and evolving relational resiliency.

Among the activities George presented, one stands out. Near the end of one of the rehearsals, group members were asked to find a partner and instructed to stand back to back. With the song "Lean on Me" playing, each pair was encouraged to literally lean on each other.[26] With separate bodies becoming one, connections between the pairs transformed from simply feeling connected to being connected. I remember very clearly the impact this exercise had on each pair when George unexpectedly stopped the music before the song had finished, likely in an attempt to end the session on time. Collectively, there was an unmistakable sense of being cheated as the group was jolted from the ephemeral experience of being in complete connection with another human being. Since that day, whenever I hear that song, I am transported back to those few minutes of being blissfully and uncomplicatedly connected to another human being.

As individuals and as a group, the company members of *Contact!Unload* were moving rapidly towards a common group membership and growth-fostering relationships that would support the difficult work ahead.

Stuck in the Middle with You: The Working Stage

The middle or working stage is the point in which the group focuses on its purpose; it is the core of the group process, whereby group members gain the most benefit from their participation.[27] Essential considerations during this stage include each member's level of participation and the degree of trust and cohesion among group members.

Looking back, three main occurrences during the development of *Contact!-Unload* characterized the trust needed throughout the working stage: 1) understanding of the veterans' experiences, 2) development and introduction of the script, and 3) group process and sharing.

Veterans' Experiences

To fully understand the veterans and their experiences, a substantial amount of time was devoted to providing a safe space for veterans to share their stories, personal truths, and experiences. As a group, the civilians took on a what David Fenell describes as a student role as we acknowledged our collective ignorance.[28] Listening with intent as we processed and held these painful narratives with compassion and awe, which Fenell states is critical in developing trust and rapport that from an RCT view, served to strengthen emerging bonds and growth-fostering relationships between the two groups.

Development and Introduction of the Script

The development of the script was vital in fortifying the veterans' trust in the project and their understanding that they had been truly heard and understood. The veterans voiced unease about how their lives would be presented and interpreted, not wanting them to be presented as, in their words, "war porn." Yet, despite these concerns, they voiced the salience of their military training and how it continued to reflect the deeply ingrained sense of honour and commitment to complete the mission. This served as a tacit reminder that intense repeated rehearsals would require significant personal sacrifice as the veterans physically and emotionally relived some of their most painful moral and psychological injuries. Doing so with a script that was subpar would have fractured the developing trust and shifting relational images, and likely would have adversely affected the upward trajectory of the still-forming superordinate group. I can only imagine the pressure lead writer Graham Lea must have felt knowing every word he scribed and every scene he developed would be evaluated, reviewed, and dissected with intense, focused scrutiny.

On the first day the script was shared, I was standing near the same veteran who flexed his ingroup muscle and roared at the civilians earlier in the group's development. As he carefully turned each page, he took off his glasses, rubbed his eyes, and gently shook his head in amazement, murmuring something along the lines of, "I can't believe he fucking got it." From this point on, it was clear to me and everyone else that the veterans were totally committed to the project.

Group Process and Sharing

For the veterans, the early days of rehearsal, like the scriptwriting phase, were filled with moments (both long and short) of anxiety, panic, overwhelming emotions, re-experiencing, heightened physiological responses, moments of dissociation, tears, and much-needed laughter to break the tension. While rehearsal was an arduous task that left the veterans emotionally, physically, spiritually, and mentally drained, they each stated that their personal suffering was worth it if it prevented even one brother or sister in arms from taking his or her life. For the civilians, there was an array of reactions, the most prominent of which was a profound sense of empathy and compassion. Unlike being able to switch TV channels or turn down the volume during the holidays when we are bombarded with commercials of suffering children, we watched the emotional and psychological suffering each veteran had been carrying play out time and time again before our very eyes.

Among the rehearsals, one stands out as being the most transformative for the entire company. After a two-week break, Marv led a group discussion and invited us to share how the project was impacting us. As each member of the group began to disclose his or her private thoughts, feelings, and experiences, it was incontrovertible that the water well of trust had surpassed the loam, sand, and gravel and was steadily seeping towards the groundwater of authentic and mutually supportive relationships. Each member was actively engaged in giving authentic feedback that enabled each of us to not only understand others in a new way but also understand how others were experiencing us as individuals.

I remember being incredibly moved as I witnessed the interpersonal risks being taken. As group members shared their individual vulnerabilities, fears, and desires, the emerging company tenderly held each person's experience and responded with accepting, thoughtful feedback. At times, I struggled to fight back the tears. To my surprise, the veteran who initially put the outgroup in their place, had reached over and was tenderly holding my hand. As I slowly turned to my right, our glassy eyes met with a synergy that manifested in reciprocal gentle and caring smiles. Divides were torn down and replaced by understanding. Acceptance and appreciation replaced rejection and mistrust. Recognizing similarities had replaced implicit and explicit differences. Group cohesion had moved beyond just being connected to one another.

Within the RCT paradigm, the level of authentic personal sharing as well as thoughtful and considered feedback enabled us as a group to experience one another in an entirely new way, a key ingredient in moving from isolation to connection.[29] These growth-fostering relationships provided a safe space for voicing personal truths in an environment that assured all of those who willingly shared that their experiences were not only important but also valued. As a group, we were becoming equal partners in a collective that was able to hold and honour each and every group member's experiences.

Every Story Has an End: Performing *Contact!Unload*

Our performances of *Contact!Unload* were the culmination of months of group building, storytelling, script development, and intensive and gut-wrenching rehearsals. Together, these experiences melded together to form a bedrock of trust that supported the entire cast and crew.

Before the Performance

The group climate leading up to each performance was marked by a collective nervousness yet also underscored individual anxieties and vulnerabilities. Even though the entire cast had similar worries about remembering lines and cues, it was clear to me as we assembled in the murk of the narrow offstage pass that the veterans shared a communal, unsettled consciousness. The consternation in their eyes said it all. They were about to publicly expose their innermost secrets and individual vulnerabilities. It was personal. It was real. Yet, despite their individual fears and anxieties, they consoled each other with firm handshakes, compassionate touches, and full embraces. Witnessing the depth of care between these men highlighted the camaraderie, friendship, appreciation, and support each had with the others, and their unique subgroup status within the company that could, and did, coexist. Although I understood that these men shared a unique bond, a small part of me was envious that I could not truly understand or be a part of that shared bond.

The civilians, on the other hand, largely kept their anxiety and concerns private. As one of the performers, however, I imagine that we shared an unspoken concern: don't screw up. We too were committed to the mission, but perhaps more importantly, we were committed to these men who had become our friends. Although it was never explicitly voiced, the veterans were depending on our precision and commitment. I was very aware that I was one of only two women in the performance representing the mothers and wives and other significant female members in the lives of our military men and women. Although this caused some anxiety, I was most anxious about 1) being part of the opening scene, unable to master marching in step with the veterans as we raised the Tribute Pole (see Chapter 6), and 2) that I was a civilian representing our female soldiers and paying homage to our fallen female troops: Nichola Kathleen Sarah Goddard, Michelle Linda Mendes, Karine Marie, Natasha Blais, and Kristal Lee-Anne Giesebrecht.

Performances

It is undeniable that the veterans' performances in *Contact!Unload* entailed unparalleled levels of vulnerability and risk. They shared parts of themselves that may not have been previously revealed to family or friends. This was further compounded by the fact that the audience represented an unknown within a larger, community group dynamic. Still, by sharing and performing their stories, the veterans had allowed themselves to be authentically seen and experienced by others, obliterating the wall of silence and moving from isolation to connection.

Throughout the three performances, the company's individual and collective roles and identities naturally oscillated. I was also acutely aware of collective shepherding among us during the performances. We held one another tight through a bottomless well of compassionate and affectionate glances, kind and thoughtful embraces, and encouraging, supportive whispers. When I cast my mind back to my own experience, something that took place during one of musician Jon Ochsendorf's soul-stirring performances stands out the most. Standing in the shadows of stage left, I was flanked by the two veterans in whose scenes I played the role of their significant other. Because of the time spent rehearsing, and our being connected by our roles, our relationships with one another was, on some level, more intimate. As the music began, we unconsciously moved closer together. I don't recall which of us reached out to touch and hold the other, but there we stood – naturally entwined, fully supported, and meaningfully connected. Viewed from an RCT framework, these intertwining, mutually respectful, growth-fostering relationships moved us as individuals and as distinct groups – from isolation to connection.

Curtain Call

During the credits that preceded the final curtain call, the company huddled together in the black of stage right. There was tension in the air. In the fleeting nanoseconds between dark that engulfed us and light that would bring us face to face with the audience, it felt like the entire company took a collective deep breath. The moment of truth was upon us – curtain call. When Graham cued the lights, the audience began applauding and, one by one, the civilians made their way onstage. The audience's anticipation of being introduced to the veterans was palpable. After the last civilian bowed and the first veteran was introduced, applause exploded. The veterans' sacrifices and experiences were validated.

Playing to three packed houses that culminated in three standing ovations was testament that the production had not only been well received but was a resounding success. These were distinctly proud moments for the entire company. Considering the veterans' misgivings about the potential negative impact and/or feedback their performances might have, their smiles and glassy eyes manifested a sense of intense pride and relief. Looking out into the audience while struggling to contain my own emotions, I began to see the audience and hear their applause as more than simply reflecting respect and admiration. To me, the audience was aching to add to the veterans' stories by letting each of them know how their stories and performances had touched them.

Post-Performance Climate
The climate after the first two performances was distinctly celebratory. Company members congratulated one another with warm embraces, kisses, handshakes, and accolades. This outpouring of authentic emotion was testament to the mutually caring, supportive, and growth-fostering relationships that had developed. Among the veterans, there were shared loving embraces born from a place of knowing what it had taken to share and perform their stories.

The natural high following these two performances was infectious, and almost everyone experienced a palpable need to be together. As a group, we descended upon local establishments to celebrate our accomplishments. During those two celebrations, there was no place for the ingroup/outgroup dynamic. We were a group of people who had moved from isolation to connection, and from connection to growth-fostering relationships. We had become friends, with developing bonds that distinctly felt like those associated with lifelong friends or the bonds often experienced with one's family of origin.

The last performance, however, marked the end of what had been an intense relational experience for everyone involved. Sitting in a circle in the middle of the theatre stage for the first of two debriefings, we were limited by the theatre's hours of operation. The natural high that characterized the earlier post-performance climate had been replaced by exhaustion, overwhelming relief, and a profound sense of sadness. Our last moments together as a company had come.

It was over. Mission accomplished.

The development and successful performances of *Contact!Unload* provided two groups of people from manifestly different cultures an opportunity to shift from a mistrustful and disconnected ingroup/outgroup dynamic to trust and connection that made space for a shared identity. Through shared experiences that promoted seeing the other in oneself, tightly held relational images of the "other" were challenged. Through risk-taking, authentic self-disclosure, and mutual empathy, feelings of safety and trust emerged as the need to overpower and dominate diminished and moved the two groups from "I" to "we." Authentic feedback shifted perspectives of the "other" and planted the seeds that grew into greater self-awareness and a more balanced view of others that enabled each of us to see the value and importance of those unlike ourselves. As a result, relational resiliency increased and culminated in the development of growth-fostering relationships that accepted and embraced the socio-cultural roles and norms that differentiate civilians from veterans. In the end, what had originated as a series of complex social phenomena with an ingroup/outgroup dynamic ended with the unchanged ingroup/outgroup dynamic that was decidedly dissimilar yet intrinsically tied to where it all began.

Final Thoughts

Civilian-Supported Veteran Transition

The idiom "If it's not broke, don't fix it" illustrates how researchers and scholars sometimes resist change and novel ideas even as new knowledge becomes available. The decision to ask civilians unknown to the veterans to be part of *Contact!Unload* illustrates how scholars can advance theory and knowledge by thinking outside the box. By moving beyond the VTN veterans-only paradigm, Marv Westwood and George Belliveau provided the four veterans with an opportunity to improve their relational resiliency and develop meaningful relationships with the largest group to which they belong – their non-military communities. When I asked one veteran what he learned from his relationships with the civilians on the project, he replied, "I am surprised how much other people really care." While there is a need and place for homogeneous veterans' groups and programs, it is important to recognize if or when homogeneity may actually thwart veteran reintegration by reinforcing a disconnection from non-military relationships as well as male-only relationships.

Women-Supported Veterans' Transition

Generally speaking, half of the world's population is made up of women, and the majority of male veterans are married to, or are in partnerships with, women. Male veterans are also likely to have multiple types of relationships with women in their roles as grandfathers, fathers, sons, brothers, uncles, friends, neighbours, and co-workers. The literature on veterans' transition clearly acknowledges relationships with spouses and families as one of the major challenges male veterans face during transition.

Considering that one of the project's goals was helping veterans increase their relational competency, the women in *Contact!Unload* played a unique role. Including women as part of the civilian group provided the veterans an opportunity to build their relational resiliency by engaging and connecting beyond how male veterans relate and communicate with one another and with other men in general. Because feedback from others is essential to self-awareness and relational growth, the feedback from women in this project provided the veterans the opportunity to develop a different type of relational resiliency through authentic engagement in platonic, mutually caring, supportive relationships. These types of experiences are important because they can foster personal insight that has the potential to shift relational images of the women in their lives. Through this, male veterans may better understand how they use or misuse power within their relationships after belonging to a culture that is male-dominated, hierarchical, and power-based.

Acknowledgments

To the veterans – Tim, Dale, Chuck, and Warren: I am honoured and privileged to be able to call each of you a friend. You informed my worldview, reminded me what bravery looks like, and modelled the importance of taking a leap of faith.

To the cast and crew of *Contact!Unload:* Thank you for your friendship and support, and for allowing me be a part of your experience.

Notes

1 B. Badenoch and P. Cox, "Integrating Interpersonal Neurobiology with Group Psychotherapy," in *Interpersonal Neurobiology of Group Psychotherapy and Group Process,* ed. B. Badenoch and S.P. Gnatt, 1–18 (London: Karnac, 2013); H.T. Reis, W.A. Collins, and E. Berscheid, "The Relationship Context of Human Behavior and Development," *Psychological Bulletin* 126, 6 (2000): 844–72.

2 D.W. Foy, S.M. Glynn, P.P. Schnurr, M.K. Jankowski, et al., "Group Therapy," in *Effective Treatments for PTSD: Practice Guidelines from the International Society for Traumatic Stress Studies,* ed. E.B. Foa, T.M. Keane, and M.J. Friedman, 155–75 (New York: Guilford, 2000); L.K. Hall, "The Importance of Understanding Military Culture," *Social Work in Health Care* 50, 1 (2011): 4–18.

3 D.L. Fenell, "Counseling Stoic Warriors: Providing Therapy to Military Men," in *A Counselor's Guide to Working with Men,* ed. M. Englar-Carlson, M.P. Evans, and T. Duffey, 227–46 (Alexandria, VA: American Counseling Association, 2014).

4 American Psychiatric Association, *Diagnostic and Statistical Manual of Mental Disorders,* 5th ed. (Washington, DC: American Psychiatric Association, 2013); C. Xue, Y. Ge, B. Tang, Y. Liu, et al., "A Meta-Analysis of Risk Factors for Combat-Related PTSD among Military Personnel and Veterans," *PLOS One* 10, 3 (2015): 1–21, https://doi.org/10.1371/journal.pone.0120270.

5 A.K. Mansfield, M.E. Addis, and W. Courtenay, "Measurement of Men's Help Seeking: Development of the Barriers to Help Seeking Scale," *Psychology of Men and Masculinity* 6, 2 (2005): 95–108.

6 V. Rozynko and H.E. Dondershine, "Trauma Focus Group Therapy for Vietnam Veterans with PTSD," *Psychotherapy: Theory, Research, Practice, Training* 28, 1 (1991): 157–61.

7 S.L. Gaertner, J.A. Mann, J.F. Dovidio, A.J. Murrell, and M. Pomare, "How Does Cooperation Reduce Intergroup Bias?" *Journal of Personality and Social Psychology* 59, 4 (1990): 692–704.

8 M.A. Hogg, "Social Categorization, Depersonalization, and Group Behavior," in *Blackwell Handbook of Social Psychology: Group Processes,* ed. M.A. Hogg and R.S. Tindale (Malden, MA: Blackwell, 2001), 56.

9 S. Gaertner, J. Dovidio, P. Anastasio, B. Bachman, and M. Rust, "The Common Ingroup Identity Model: Recategorization and the Reduction of Intergroup Bias," *European Review of Social Psychology* 4, 1 (1993): 1–26.

10 Ibid.

11 J.B. Miller, *Toward a New Psychology of Women* (Boston: Beacon, 1986).

12 V. Bryson, *Feminist Political Theory: An Introduction,* 2nd ed. (New York: Palgrave Macmillan, 2003).

13 J.V. Jordan, *Relational-Cultural Therapy* (Washington, DC: American Psychological Association, 2010); T. Duffey and S. Haberstroh, "Developmental Relational Counseling: Applications for Counseling Men," *Journal of Counseling and Development* 92, 1 (2014): 104–13.

14 J.V. Jordan, "The Role of Mutual Empathy in Relational/Cultural Therapy," *Journal of Clinical Psychology* 56, 8 (2000): 1005–16; Jordan, *Relational-Cultural Therapy.*

15 Badenoch and Cox, "Integrating Interpersonal Neurobiology with Group Psychotherapy"; L.J. Cozolino, *The Neuroscience of Human Relationships: Attachment and the Developing Social Brain,* 2nd ed. (New York: Norton, 2014).

16 Jordan, *Relational-Cultural Therapy.*

17 J.V. Jordan and L.M. Hartling, "New Developments in Relational-Cultural Theory," in *Rethinking Mental Health and Disorders: Feminist Perspectives,* ed. M. Ballou and L.S. Brown (New York: Guilford, 2002), 54.

18 Jordan, *Relational-Cultural Therapy;* Jordan, "The Role of Mutual Empathy in Relational/Cultural Therapy."

19 Jordan, *Relational-Cultural Therapy.*

20 Duffey and Haberstroh, "Developmental Relational Counseling."

21 Ibid.

22 Ibid., 109.

23 E.E. Jacobs, R.L. Masson, R.L. Harvill, and C.J. Schimmel, *Group Counseling: Strategies and Skills,* 7th ed. (Belmont, CA: Brooks/Cole-Thomson Learning, 2012).

24 M.J. Westwood and P. Wilensky, *Therapeutic Enactment: Restoring Vitality through Trauma Repair in Groups* (Vancouver: Group Action Press, 2005).

25 Ibid.

26 B. Withers, vocal performance of "Lean on Me," by Bill Withers, released April 21, 1972, on *Still Bill,* Sussex, 33⅓ rpm.

27 Jacobs et al., *Group Counseling.*

28 Fenell, "Counseling Stoic Warriors."

29 Jordan, *Relational-Cultural Therapy.*

13

Contact!Unload Revisited
Degrees of Separation

Lynn Fels

I am an innocent bystander.
I don't want to be implicated.
What connection do I have with Afghanistan?

June 16th, 6:12 pm, 2016

Bicycling over Burrard Street Bridge in Vancouver, I summon up all the possible connections I have with a war that was fought in a country beyond the boundaries of my imagination.

A setting sun reflects multiple faces in multiple office tower windows.

Six degrees of separation –

My maternal grandfather fought in the First World War, *a war to end all wars.*
Nineteen, he caught pneumonia in the trenches in France, and was decommissioned.
His escape made possible the birth of my mother, my birth.

My paternal grandfather was a major in the Second World War.
He converted, so that his papers wouldn't betray his Jewish heritage.

My cousin's stepson signed up for Afghanistan. A reserve officer, he believed he couldn't in good conscience train soldiers to go overseas if he had never been himself.

I mailed handwritten letters to my nephew at boot camp.
I wrote about the cottage, swimming, and canoeing, but not of my fear for him.

Roshan Thomas, for whom I, and others, had failed to create a Canadian International Development Agency research project in support of her school for girls, was killed in a restaurant in Kabul.

Not six degrees –

◇◇◇◇◇◇◇

June 16th, 6:43 pm, 2016

Locking my bike to a bicycle rack, I take a breath, feel a summer breeze, and then head into an office building. "Studio's in the basement." The elevator doors open to an empty corridor. A janitor points the way to Foster Eastman's studio. I have been invited to a reading of *Contact!Unload*, my third encounter with the play, having seen a rehearsal, and a full performance at Granville Island a year earlier. At the door of the studio, Dr. Marv Westwood greets me, gesturing with his hand, "Follow me, I want you to see this." He leads me past the studio out to the back of the building where they are filming a soldier who is answering questions about the art he has just created by shooting paint with an assault rifle at a faceless outline of a soldier.[1] The audio technician motions us to silence.

Why did you aim the gun at the heart?
Why did you choose those particular colours?
What do they mean to you?

I look at the panels where violence, pain, memory, hope, release streak colours of paint down outlined bodies of faceless soldiers. Graphic art.

"I'm going to create a panel for each one of the soldiers who died," whispers the artist. Another soldier steps forward to the microphone.

A fake AK-47 lies on the cement floor.
Too close to the Orlando massacre.[2] Too close to home.

April 30, 2015, 19:45

I am aware of tension, a crisis, behind the scenes. The performance is delayed. I sit in the dark as minutes tick relentlessly. There is no recapturing time.

Guitar chords sound, a voice enters through darkness,
and I fall into the lyrics of loss –

a black sedan[3]

ATTENTION! QUICK MARCH! LEFT, RIGHT, LEFT, RIGHT![4]

   Two coffins, attached end to end, the names of the 158 Canadian soldiers killed in Afghanistan carved into the wood, await the arrival of the actors. Boots drum the beat as soldiers march onstage. Pallbearers. You can feel the burden in the silence between footsteps. They lift, then raise the coffins upright into position, arms above heads, hand over hand, muscles straining. A Tribute Pole.

And watching, I am reminded of the Iwo Jima memorial statue of six American soldiers carrying forth the American flag that called soldiers into battle. Did the director foresee the symbolism, the echoing of a past war, in the staging of this scene? A comparative moment that evokes the endless repetition of war, a statue of a moment frozen in bronze, urging others to victory, and here, a living tribute enacted, the weight of war and death carried and raised, for those who have fallen, hands touching names of dead buddies?

I keep a breath's distance, attending to the play with a critic's eye, to protect the thin veil between what is shared onstage and my responsibility to watch, to listen. This witnessing is not without uneasiness.

I carry the burden of being present.

Confession. Veil is not my word, but borrowed from a soldier who DEMANDED, during the talkback after the play's reading a year later, that counsellors listening to stories such as those revealed onstage should STOP HIDING behind veils. The veils they raise between themselves and those who are wounded, lost, without hope, in despair, sitting with them in their counselling offices, behind closed doors.

My veil is unraveling,
stitch by stitch
revealing a wound
        unsuspected, not-yet known.

June 16th, 8:35 pm, 2016

Boredom.

Soldiers waiting –
    in the heat of the moment, in fear, in anticipation
poised between boredom, action, death, survival –

VET 2: There'd be days of boredom. Weeks of boredom.

VET 3: Starin' out at a desert that never fucking changes.

VET 2: I've watched that same rock for days.

Imagine being trapped in boredom interrupted by bursts of gunfire –

I sit on the rug in Foster's studio as the play's reading unfolds. Not so much a reading, but a re-enactment, bodies pace into the light, into audience space. The divide between us is ill-defined. No fourth wall. Surrounding us, in midst of the action, is Foster's art; records drip red. Toilet seats intertwined overhead. Faceless soldiers on panels. Art that doesn't permit a moment or space to breathe. No glass of white wine to ease tense nerves, we are going commando this evening –

VET 3: You wait. Wait for those seconds, minutes, those moments.

VET 2: That's what you wait for.

VET 3: Not your family ... over here they can't exist ...

VET 2: They can't exist or you die.

VET 3: So, you wait to get shot. Wait to see if you're going to –

Unable to see the performers, I inch closer, wanting to see their faces, their bodies – a voyeur eager to see the damage of what happens when something blows up – like when I watched the television camera trained on a hut in the Iraqi desert as we waited for an airplane to bomb the enemy hidden inside. The plane arrives, but the cameraman jostles the camera as he leaps to safety; all I can see is a blue sky askew. And then, humiliation, shame, to understand that I am a spectator, capable and culpable of turning war into entertainment, wanting to see behind the curtain, into the place of killing.

I tell no one, then everyone. The shock and shame and hunger of wanting to watch ...

And into boredom CONTACT! ENGAGE! ENGAGE! ENGAGE! automatic fire erupts. Who?! What?! Where?! Where? What! Who?!

Startled out of my skin, out of complacency, what the –

EXPLOSION!

Get out of the vehicle, try to save his ass there's blood everywhere sweating putting quick clot on him burns your hands fuck, it's horrible helicopter flying around somewhere with some goddammed general I hope you like your fucking flight should be my friend on that helicopter ...

I lean in, barely breathing, I lean in, as soldiers bend over the injured soldier, as they draw together in a frozen tableau. Michelangelo's *Pieta,* the

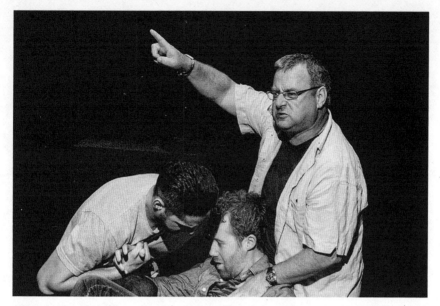

Figure 21 Leaning over the body of a soldier. Left to right: Phillip Lopresti, Oliver Longman, and Chuck MacKinnon | Photo by Blair McLean; used with permission.

mother of Jesus, weeps over her dead son; here onstage, in the reading, in the field, soldiers lean over the body of a soldier.

(Here is a statue they will not commission an artist to render.)

In, out. In, out. Come on breathe motherfucker. Nothin' I could do. Put his head on my lap, my hand right there I could feel his breath. In and out, and in and out. Gettin' shallow. Tried to tell him I ... I ... I told him it shoulda been me. Shoulda ... In and out, and in and out and ... and ...
(Beat)
Despair, horror, grief, rage.
It shoulda been me.

Chopper finally comes. Put him on a stretcher and load him in. Fucking stretcher wouldn't fit in the goddam fucking helicopter. Couldn't close the fucking door. Had to tip him out inside the ... fucking blood everywhere. Last thing I saw was the soles of his boots.

Last thing I saw was the soles of his boots.

Souls. Lost souls.

I weep.
Bastards. I am on the front line.

The impact of the reading of the play in the artist's studio was unanticipated.

Invited guests. A room full of counsellors. Food and music. A man with a guitar. Theatre awaits an audience. Released, theatre can catch you unawares. Raw. Flesh flayed. Script interrupted. I am compromised. The studio was where work on the play with the soldiers, the veterans, had originally unfolded, along with the carving of the Tribute Pole – echoes revisited. The space is haunted, vibrates with an energy that strips us naked.

A wound that refuses to heal.

You cannot escape the dark, the noise, the pain, the unfolding embodied telling of grief that holds you rigid, afraid to speak; to lean into the action is to lose balance, to fall into yourself, with no hands to guide you to a gentle landing. In the telling, the wound is revealed.

158 Canadian soldiers killed in battle.
We do not count the suicides on home ground.

> 158 Canadian soldiers died in the Afghanistan mission. But the losses do not end there. A *Globe and Mail* investigation reveals a disturbing number the military has kept secret: that at least 54 soldiers and vets killed themselves after they returned from war.
>
> – *The Globe and Mail*, Feb. 23, 2016, 10:14 am[5]

Okay. Wait a second. I don't get it.
PTSD I get ... sure. Lots of press on that!
I've read the articles.
Depression?

Well yes, no surprise, it's hell over there
and not so great coming back –

But suicide as a war casualty?

Who you gonna tell ...?
Who wants to listen ...?

Suicide because ...

If I speak he'll –
If I speak she'll –

Mental illness as a war injury?

He got home safe, didn't she?[6]

FATHER: It's just as terrible as dying from a bomb or a bullet. No, it's crueler. Takes longer to kill.

BROTHER: It's more vicious. Gets inside ya. Gets inside all of us.

Theatre dwells in ambiguity, opens what is not yet known, invites meaning-making, brings into clarity that which is not yet recognized. Three-dimensional action witnessed disrupts two-dimensional thinking. Time interrupts. Drags you forward and backwards.

A soldier killed in Afghanistan, his only brother disappears days later during a camping trip. I saw the headline.[7] Missing. Still missing. Watching the performers onstage, listening to their words, brings home what has been a half-understood connection.

Collateral damage happens within families
                                         within communities ...

Mental illness as a casualty of war.
We have been careless. Are we still counting ...?

Headlines read in newspapers, when replayed through living bodies, expose stories lived that are visceral, unveiled, offered as an opportunity to us, as audience, as witness, to learn, to dwell within the unimaginable, unsayable, unspeakable. Metaphors, symbols, interrupt everyday meaning-making to create new understandings. At home, I can turn the page of the newspaper, switch off the radio, click off the TV screen. Unless I leave the theatre, I cannot avoid its offering.

The lines of the script are not contained within the script. Pre-performance, post-performance, actions evoke actions, words spoken, relationships navigate difficult territories, contact made, cracks open, reveal light, shadows.

Be careful of the post-performance blues.

I hate you! I hate you! I hate you!
   Yet I must do this in remembrance of you who are not here.
I must do this in the hope of you who are yet to arrive.

An unexpected stranger has entered the space. Pulsing through the veins of the men who are sitting present before us. Post-performance. Here is the injury of war. Here is the injury of us. Here is a wound that refuses to heal. To heal is to forget.

A soldier confesses that, on coming home, he had thought that nobody cared. Silence makes us complicit.

◇◇◇◇◇◇

DALE: (*pointing to a bracelet on his wrist*) That is a band of brothers (*Female vet beside DALE elbows him gently*) and of sisters. That is why we fought. That's why we keep fighting. And we're still a band. We're still bound.

DALE: He knows that I will die for him, and I know that he will die for me.

The unspoken bond between soldiers is impenetrable, unbreakable, recognized but unknown to others, the burden, the weight, the promise.

How unbearable to learn when you are fighting for each other's lives, that another soldier has taken his life –

One, two, three, four –
      When does the dying end?

And here is the line in the play, in life, in reflection that troubles. Reading the notes of the play, now in this writing, there is another possible understanding.

June 16th, 10:45, 2016

I bicycle home in anger
Along West Georgia Street over the Burrard Street Bridge
I rage about the injury done to me, unforewarned
these stories bludgeon
victim on the front line, how will I sleep tonight?

There could have been notice of counsellors available in the room, as is often done during introductions to forum theatre for public audiences.

But I knew the counsellors in the room, by name, by reputation, colleagues, friends ...

What tears, what questions, I wonder, are they now grappling with in their drive home? What guilt?

The revealing of these stories, through theatre, through the retelling,
are wounding,
re-wounding those who tell, those who listen.

A burden, this telling of woundedness and unresolved pain.

 A long ride home, along the curve of the ocean, by Kitsilano beach, and anger dissipates. To be made uneasy is the responsibility, the art of theatre; to shake someone awake, to call us to attention.

"Listen, I must tell you my story, in the best way I can.

I'm bleeding all over the place. What are you going to do?"

Dear Member of Parliament,
I don't want Canada to participate in war.
I don't want Canada to sell armoured vehicles to Saudi Arabia.
 I don't want Canada to be a country that sells or buys weapons.
 I want my Canada to stand on guard for peace in peace.

I want my Canada to be a haven of forgiveness, opportunity, renewal.

I want our country to take care of our soldiers.

In the Second World War, the soldiers returned to benefits for homes, education, opportunities for jobs, life-long pensions for the injured.

Meaningful work.

Contact!Unload has woken me up. I am responsible for the story behind the headlines.

◇◇◇◇◇◇◇

Chuck,[8] I would tell you this in person, but I can't because I cry just in the remembering.

I do not have your courage to speak to my truth.

To be wounded again and again and again and again and again and again ...

And yet you insist. You will not be quiet. You are a play within a play within a play within the presence of our not listening.
My refusal to listen. My fear to listen.

A boy incinerated, wheeled into camp in a wheelbarrow.
What we don't talk about.

Here is the secret hidden between the lines of the play.
The unspoken, the unsayable, the unsaid.[9]
The gap between –

hundreds of little graves

Here is what I refuse to see. My responsibility. My complicity.

◇◇◇◇◇◇◇

Now I know what I could have told you.

> *In the Prince George airport, passengers are hustling, bustling, drinking coffee, impatiently checking their cell phones. The waiting room is crowded, Sunday evening, everyone is travelling home somewhere else. First, Air Canada announces a delay in departure. Five minutes later, WestJet echoes the announcement. A soccer game plays on the screens overhead. A plane sits on the tarmac, its doors remain shut. You can taste confusion in the air. A white plane appears on the horizon, angles towards Earth, wheels kiss the tarmac, rolls to a stop. I watch as the airplane hatch door opens, passengers file down the stairs, lugging carry-ons, vanish out of sight.*
>
> *I am drawn to the window in curiosity, a black sedan drives into view, brakes slowly to a stop. Soldiers march in formation, in uniform. A family*

stands on the tarmac, arms around waists, hands clasped, and still I don't understand.

The cargo door opens, the luggage ramp positioned.
And then,
a solitary coffin descends.
A plate glass window separates me from Afghanistan.
I watch as the coffin is received by the pallbearers, carried and placed with care, tenderly, into the back of the sedan, the hearse drives away at a funereal pace, followed by the soldiers, followed by the bereaved family, who have welcomed home a son, a brother, a fallen comrade. Dead.

A silence behind me, so deep, it weighs on my shoulders, and I turn. Standing, all of us are standing, silent, called into the moment by death, by ritual, in sorrow, in respect of a young man's life lost. Two planeloads of passengers, mothers, fathers, brothers, sisters, sons, daughters, aunts, uncles, nieces, nephews, grandparents, arrested, all had risen, as I stood watching out the window, and witnessed a soldier's arrival home. The sight stole my breath away and touched my heart – we care.

There are moments when we cannot speak to the heart loss within.

And yet we must.

I am sorry

I am not an innocent bystander.

I am complicit.

I am present.

I'll live for you if you live for me.

Acknowledgments

I would like to thank Drs. Marv Westwood and George Belliveau for their invitation to participate in the project as an audience member. My heartfelt appreciation for the learning offered me by the soldiers and veterans whose work is embedded within the play, and to Dr. Graham Lea for his permission to use excerpts from the original play in this writing. And my thanks especially to Chuck, who graced us with the cracks of his world, within which I glimpsed a light.

Notes

1 The painting was part of the creation of the SERIOUSshit art project. See Chapter 6.
2 This refers to the killing and wounding of dozens of patrons in a gay nightclub in Orlando, Florida, on June 12, 2016, which occurred just prior to the reading. See L. Alvarez, R.

Pérez-Penà, and C. Hauser, "Orlando Gunman Was 'Cool and Calm' after Massacre, Police Say," *New York Times,* June 13, 2016, http://www.nytimes.com/2016/06/14/us/orlando-shooting.html.

3 Musician Jon Ochsendorf provided music throughout the original performance of *Contact!Unload.* The show began with his song "Black Sedan," which tells the story of a family hoping they never see the black sedan come to their door carrying news of the death of their son in Afghanistan.

4 Extracts from the play *Contact!Unload* are inserted throughout, courtesy of the playwright, Dr. Graham Lea. An italicized portion of the script has been changed to present tense, with extracts from the script following, interspersed (but not identified) with the writer's text to complete the scene. Excerpts are from Moment 1, Moment 5, Moment 8, Moment 12, and Moment 19.

5 R. D'Aliesio, "The Unremembered," *Globe and Mail,* February 23, 2016, http://www.theglobeandmail.com/news/veterans/article26499878/.

6 The gender shifts to acknowledge that Canadian women also fought in Afghanistan.

7 This incident was reported by the *Globe and Mail:* A. Ligaya, "Brother of Dead Soldier Missing in B.C. Interior," *Globe and Mail,* July 24, 2007, http://www.theglobeandmail.com/news/national/brother-of-dead-soldier-missing-in-bc-interior/article689810/.

8 One of the veterans. See Chapter 2.

9 On trauma and witnessing, see J. Salverson, "Taking Liberties: A Theatre Class of Foolish Witnesses," *Research in Drama Education* 13, 2 (2008): 245–55.

14
Remembering

Carl Leggo

IN ANTHONY DOERR'S NOVEL *All the Light We Cannot See,* the narrator notes that "it's embarrassingly plain how inadequate language is."[1] Doerr's narrative, located in France during the Second World War, presents a harrowing account of destruction, deprivation, and death while also evoking an abiding sense of human commitment to hope, beauty, memory, and love. While writers readily understand the truism that language is inadequate, writers also know that when language is rendered creatively with both artful and heartful attention to story making, language can also move us to imaginative and empathetic understandings of living experiences. And in turn, language can transform us.

When I sat in the audience for a performance of *Contact!Unload,* I witnessed the creative confluence of military veterans, scholars, educators, actors, musicians, and artists as they remembered the complex stories of war, investigated the psychic wounds of memory, and supported one another with courage and love to tell the stories that are almost impossible to share. In their eloquent and brave performance, the cast of *Contact!Unload* sang out the almost unspeakable because they knew that speaking the stories was integral to health and hope, because they understood that many people needed to hear and know the stories.

My father-in-law, whom I call Pop, was almost ninety-one years old when I first saw *Contact!Unload.* I met Pop when I was sixteen years old – I had just begun dating his daughter. Pop has been like a father for more than forty-seven years. I have grown up with him; he has been one of my significant teachers. He is a veteran of the Second World War. He was deployed to Italy as a member of the Royal Newfoundland Regiment. A few months ago, he acknowledged that he could no longer live in the house he had known as home for almost four decades. He made plans to move to the Department of Veterans Affairs (DVA) wing of the local assisted care facility. He was informed that the DVA wing was currently full, but he could move to another wing of the facility and perhaps move again to the DVA wing when a room became available. My father-in-law said simply, "If a room is not available in the DVA, I won't go." Later, he explained that he wanted to spend his last days with the men he had known since he was a young recruit in the army. "We look out for one another," he added. Some weeks later, a DVA room became available, and Pop moved. He now plays cards with Bob, who was a sergeant in the Regiment. Pop says daily, "I feel at home here. I am content." More than seventy years have passed since Pop fought in the Second World War, and even after all those years, in this last chapter of his life, he wants to be with other veterans. He knows they will look out for one another. As he anticipates the end of his long life, he looks to his buddies to come alongside. As they always have.

At the end of Anthony Doerr's novel, one of the main characters, Marie-Laure, reflects on her life from the perspective of the turn from the twentieth century to the twentieth-first century. Marie-Laure was a young woman during the Second World War. Now an elderly woman, she thinks: "Every hour ... someone for whom the war was memory falls out of the world. We rise again in the grass. In the flowers. In songs."[2] How do we remember? How do we challenge the loss of memory? We remember by telling stories, lots of stories. *Contact!Unload* tells the stories, and it tells the stories in drama, music, art, poetry, and performance so we can know. And while we can know only a little of the horror of war, we can know enough to know that we must always honour the men and women who protect us, the women and men who fight on our behalf, the men and women who embody our hopes.

Remembering
(for Pop)

he is at home in the circle of storytellers
always sure the story never ends

he has lived much of his life
with a bemused patience

like the world is not exactly
what he was expecting but

it has proven to be a lot
better than it might be

he has always moved deliberately
like he knows he will arrive without rushing

the greatest gift he offers
is his love, lived daily with hope

and in loving us, he teaches us,
still, how to love and live

On July 1, 2016, Pop joined other military veterans to greet Princess Anne, Queen Elizabeth II's daughter, in Corner Brook, Newfoundland. Princess Anne is the Colonel-in-Chief of the Royal Newfoundland Regiment. July 1, 2016, marked one hundred years since the most horrendous military battle in Newfoundland's history – long remembered as the battle of Beaumont-Hamel.

Still Remembering

A cold Canada Day, 2016, we huddled
at the Bay of Islands War Memorial
to remember soldiers who died,
July 1, 1916, so long ago, like it
might be yesterday. Thirty-three years
before becoming a Canadian province,
Newfoundland lived one of its darkest tales:
the first day of the Battle of the Somme
when the Royal Newfoundland Regiment
saw faraway Beaumont-Hamel in France.
The order was given to go over the top.
The Newfoundland soldiers had to cross
230 metres of barren ground raked
with German gunfire before they could
even reach their own front line. The soldiers
never stood a chance. In less than an hour,
255 men died, 386 more were wounded,
and 91 others were simply unaccounted for.
The next morning, only 68 men answered
roll call. Every Newfoundland officer
was killed or wounded. The British divisional
commander later wrote: *It was a magnificent*
display of trained and disciplined valour,
and its assault failed of success only
because dead men can advance no further.

I was much moved by the performance of *Contact!Unload* – a testimony to courage, a refutation to forgetting, a witness to remembering. May every day be a day of remembering! May our remembering be filled with thanksgiving!

Notes

1 A. Doerr, *All the Light We Cannot See* (New York: Scribner, 2014), 503.
2 Ibid., 529.

15

A Poet(h)ic Reflection on *Contact!Unload*
Voices of Women through War

Heather Duff

Like a Desert Flower

Like a desert flower waiting for rain,
like a riverbank thirsting for the touch of pitchers,
like the dawn
longing for light,
and like a house,
like a house in ruins for want of a woman –
the exhausted ones of our times
need a moment to breathe,
need a moment to sleep,
in the arms of peace, in the arms of peace.

– Parween Faiz Zadah Malaal[1]

IT WAS A HAPPY STUMBLING upon "Like a Desert Flower" by the Afghan woman poet Parween Faiz Zadah Malaal (2013). This poem resonates with my intent as I respond poet(h)ically[2] to the groundbreaking research-based play about Canadian soldiers in Afghanistan and their subsequent return as veterans. In my original poem following, cited lines are indented to act as reference points and prompts, as I respond to the gestalt of the play. I inquire in tribute to unheard women's voices, impressions and feminine imagery, my imagined layer beneath powerful stories of the aftermath of war dramatized in *Contact!Unload*. Karen Meyer contends that language includes "not only the spoken, but also the unspeakable, and the silence of the unsaid."[3] I struggle poet(h)ically with a language of silence in relation to womenfolk connected to the veterans' dramatized story; only a small number of women are featured in the play. Two female actors play supporting or minor characters in *Contact!Unload*. I find myself longing to make them more real, although few are known to the audience except

TIM's girlfriend; her disembodied if innocent voice echoes from the back of the audience, asking TIM, the recovering veteran, if he would like to attend a movie with her. After her first invitation, TIM tells her to "F– off." In the last scene, TIM surrenders by accepting her invitation, which actualizes his healing shift, and thus the research-based play concludes on a note of hope.[4] Another female actor on stage throughout – as both a literal and symbolic presence of women in service – plays in a scene featuring the bereaved mother of a returned soldier who suffered from depression.[5] At one point, this actor, playing a soldier, jokingly challenges gendered military discourse.[6]

Arguably, men's mental health is intrinsically linked to women's mental health. If we strive to address and prioritize critical ethical issues around the recovery of Canadian veterans, we ought to look equally towards women's voices linked to a necessary healing across war narratives – towards women's unique perspectives, languages, and stories. Veterans Affairs Canada offers resources such as "Lest We Forget Her," lesson plans for educators and anecdotal stories by Canadian women involved directly in wartime history.[7] In more recent times, Canadians honour military heroines such as Nichola Goddard, the first Canadian woman to die in combat.[8] Canadians are encouraged to respect and honor women's right to share equally in soldiering.[9] Growing media attention focuses specifically, however, on the immediate and post-traumatic scars of sexual harassment and assault for Canadian women in the military.[10] Many of these women fight private battles for personal safety amid the military hierarchy, posing an additional arena of brokenness unique to Canadian women soldiers and veterans. Women are included as service members in the veterans' healing community. There may be an ethical gap in this area, however, as the transition to civilian life makes more visible another layer of marginalized voices and narratives. Arguably, more research is needed towards developing strategies for healing, emancipation, and justice, particularly for women serving in the Canadian military, as well as for those women linked to veterans through family ties.

From a literary criticism perspective, Donna Coates identifies authors such as Nellie McClung, L.M. Montgomery, and others, whose fictional female characters struggle with their roles in wartime, often adopting "militaristic language as a strategy for overcoming oppression."[11] Coates contends that "Canadian women writers may seem to be speaking the same language as men, but in using the masculine colloquy of war, they are not reproducing the same history, not replicating stories already written by the dominant ideology."[12]

My poet(h)ic response to the uniqueness of women's experience of war is expressed through the genre of poetry. In the world of my original poem, "Tomb" is a meta-fictional name for the unknown soldier's wife – sometimes a wife in letter and other times a wife in spirit. Through curriculum scholar Ted Aoki's notion of *hito*, or self-other, we glean an Eastern wisdom that self and other are two equal parts of the same Japanese word.[13] Related to *hito*, Karen Meyer writes about the importance of four notions – time, place, self, and other – whereby "self and place are inextricably connected as are identity and home."[14] We may envision healing not only locally but on a global scale across a shared human history of "wars and rumours of wars."[15] We may boldly disrupt the field of mental health with respect to a gendered awareness of various forms, manifestations, and metaphors of soldiering – in far-off places, on home soil, and in places in between, where memory lingers, possesses, or haunts. We may need to claim a transcending self/other respect that knows no borders, that knows a breath of peaceful spaces where redemptivity may be realized even if in a temporal or tentative way. I recall these lines from "Like a Desert Flower":

the exhausted ones of our times
need a moment to breathe[16]

The notion of the "unknown soldier" may point to a truth beyond the notion of a soldier who died without anyone knowing his name, as there are many ways to feel nameless. War ought not to exist, but it does. The "unknown" may also reflect the ambiguity of an indefinable wound of war within individual, domestic, and community spheres. Gaps in family, community, and global recovery from violent trauma seem to be endless as full-colour news segments depicting people's response to senseless violence grace our television sets. We are left wondering about the efficacy of all those candlelit vigils. From the perspective of life-wounded soldiers, their families, and descendants representing a panoply of vital cultures, a question emerges: how, then, can we know truth between fleeting breaths of peace? Can truth be known, in the watering of the parched places?

Tomb, the Unknown Soldier's Wife

We were asked to do something disruptive in the field of men's mental health.

Starin' out at a desert that never fucking changes. I've watched that same rock for days. You wait. Wait for those seconds, minutes, those moments. Not for your family ... over here they can't exist. They can't exist, or you die ... So, you wait to get shot. Wait to see if you're going to –

– MOMENT 5

I

In Afghanistan, dryer red-white sands drift
sand the face of an angel, a figment, or pink desert primrose
by a rock-shield that blooms in particles of dust.

Tomb is a trace of imagined breeze
blister in heat, rosary of sweat beads around your neck
or tasbih: names of God, ninety and nine.

Arthritic trigger finger runs through vacant carpal tunnels,
someone's racing heart, your own, death wish
in flare of sun, only to strike love's memory the whole war,

and all history.

You are the unwelcome soldier, a waking dream,
arid fantasy, endorphins, psychosis: you watch
for valid proof of existence, for a feminine face of God.

You watch yourself wait for the next gunfire
while a scorched acacia tree in silhouette
waits for cease fire under her demure shade.

Tomb is an empty clay vessel of mirage water
in withered expanse far from home
on the empty bridge between life-death,

sans language, sans silence, "sans teeth ... sans everything"[17]
all emotion and memory enjoyed in time's fraction
and surprise about breath and another,

breath, breathed.

Tomb, a common swear word hurled
into the darkness: boomerang, flash memory
of silken cries, from your laundry bag pillow ...

vacant wet dream in chill of early dawn in the base
a silence everyone hears,
the cool, faceless, twisted aftermath

of an unexpected bomb.

Pause. It is friendly fire.

(we believe if we say the "F" word enough times,
pain will

dissipate).

II

It is a new desert for her, life alone.

Here there are no soldiers.
Here there are no boyfriends, no husbands.
We wait for life.

Tomb waits behind an ironing board, presses cream sheets
"redundant housework," her mother would say;
she irons, precise, the way her grandmother once did,
for their love nest where, at least, she can
make a shape of angel wings
between fresh cream-coloured cotton.

Her Canadian three-year-old,
playing USA helicopter,
falls "dead" crying out in the next room.

That man overseas, wandering the desert
like some crazed Old Testament character
armed with artillery, tempted by sunlit water,
the mesmerizing glare of a middle Eastern sun,

rays hot with unfriendly fire.

Tomb, the unknown soldier's wife, has no lines
except the lines she inherits from
the frayed hem of her denim skirt.

She wants to write her own lines, to be in this play

but there is no paper. She looks everywhere
for a scrap of paper.

Instead, the man's face, shaved military clean
comes home, as generations of soldiers' wives
have waited for return of hearts, over-beating
or no hearts, or dead men, or men you don't know anymore,
her pixie scent, forgotten or remembered.

Back home, she is a sounding board,
a rendering, vessel of emptied water in a
scorched land, only listen to what is unsaid.

He looks different, she muses, older, talks different.
She wonders if it is the same man from her wedding photo
or a government-sponsored imposter.

Back in the desert, soldiers defended
something spurious, ephemeral; they reached
hands into each other's wounds, doubting

Tomb places her fingers there, too ... He winces.

Idea for a painting: the waterless places?

I'd hate for anyone I love to have a look inside my head.

— DALE, *CONTACT!UNLOAD*, MOMENT 10

III

Blois, France, 1948
That old postcard: 18th century stone bridge, o'er the Loire,
eleven elliptical arches rise from the river, where,
with current, wild ducks wind through the arches.

From her casement window in 1814,
Napoleon's second wife: Marie Louise[18]
would have watched villagers trudge
over that bridge, with carts, dogs, dribbling milk buckets.

It's still there, Blois, after centuries of wars:
even Jeanne d'Arc in 1429,[19]
asks the Archbishop's blessing, before driving
those damned English from Orléans;
crafted leather, their curled boot steps,

over an older bridge, forerunner to the one I stand on.

I listen to Jeanne listen, ethereal voices
calling from the spaces between rowboats
by the river Loire, at Blois
to lick, crackle, and choke of the vision fire.

Blois, France, 1976
My oldest friend and I, stand on the bridge at Blois,
clutches her grandfather's sepia post–World War II postcard.
The Bridge at Blois, she reads. We hold it up to match.
"Now we are in the postcard," I say.

He asked us to find her.

Tomb is a memory of a mistress in France
an unknown soldier's wife, with no certificate
no deed to a house, no future nor past.

She is beautiful – dark chestnut eyes, and laugh like an April waterfall;
she laughs more than a wife in Canada,
laughs entre shell fire, among sandbag sofas
her French bread, hand-baked,
still scorching hot from a clay oven,
drips with hand-churned butter and kisses like the
moist white light of a near-death experience;
she wears what no Canadian wife can know
black sheer stockings and silk garters,
not sold back home in those general stores
where even sugar is rationed,
where you can twist your soul
those winding tornado roads of rural Ontario.

How can we look her up from a 1940's postcard
with no return address, and a fountain pen signature,
wrinkled and blurred with tears?

We will tell my friend's grandfather
she died and we found her tombstone.
Jolie. Non. *Annette.* Mais, non. *Margaux, Olivie, Renée.*

We will tell him the truth, that we saw the bridge again,
at least we saw that bridge
but we didn't see her; we are so very sorry,
but we couldn't find her.

IV

> *D'you even see what we were shooting? ... Do you think it might have been friendlies?*
>
> *All I saw was dust?*
>
> *Yeah, that's all your girlfriend sees is dust.*
>
> – VETERANS, *CONTACT!UNLOAD*, MOMENT 5

Tomb, the unknown soldier's wife,
lives in assorted waterless places.

She is wife of refugees, mother of children
with new Canadian passports,
the expectant click of their spines broken open
and stamped with fresh ink,

she is mother of anyone's child, her own, yours,
children of schoolyards, foster homes, waterfront mansions,
corporate Christmas parties, dens of iniquity,
soundless hunger cries.

Don't worry. This is friendly fire.

Tomb asks the personified windowpane:
how can fire be friendly?
as she looks out, streetlamps dim
as a summer rain-drenched alley
pours brown rivulets into a sewer
while, aka "foxtail lilies,"
three giant desert candles bloom tall
white and stately in her rented suite garden –
(some botanical fluke in the rainforest)
near blue recycled boxes overturned
and by artful crows, food scraps and packaging
strewn like rotting confetti
adorn her query: "*Is there forgiveness?*"

Pigeons, like a row of soldiers on a telephone wire:
I know. Make a peace.

Notes

1 Reproduced from *Prairie Schooner*, 87, 4 (winter 2013), by permission of the University of Nebraska Press.
2 Poet(h)ic inquiry is a pedagogical space of inquiry at the confluence of playwriting, ethics, and spirit, in the context of research-based theatre. This approach offers ethical reflection incorporating poetic-aesthetic values in arts-based research through playwriting in research-based theatre. H. Duff, "Visiting Griffin at the Confluence of Playwriting, Ethics, and Spirit: Towards Poet(h)ic Inquiry in Research-Based Theatre" (PhD dissertation, University of British Columbia, 2016), https://open.library.ubc.ca/collections/ubctheses/24/items/1.0315366.
3 K. Meyer, "Living Inquiry: Me, My Self and Other," *Journal of Curriculum Theorizing* 26, 1 (2010): 86, https://journal.jctonline.org/index.php/jct/article/view/150/64.
4 See Moment 3 and the end of Moment 21 in the Annotated Playscript in this volume.
5 The original version of Moment 12 featured a FATHER and MOTHER character. The MOTHER was adapted to UNCLE in later versions of the script.
6 See Moment 19.
7 "Canada Remembers Women in the Canadian Military," Veterans Affairs Canada, November 28, 2017, https://www.veterans.gc.ca/eng/remembrance/those-who-served/women-veterans/military.

8 V. Fortney, "In Afghanistan, Canada's Female Soldiers Earned the Right to Fight, and Die, as Equals," Canada.com, February 28, 2012, http://www.canada.com/health/Afghanistan+Canada+female+soldiers+earned+right+fight+equals/6191423/story.html; S. Goddard, *Canada's Daughter: The Story of Captain Nichola Goddard* (Belfast, PE: Underhill Books, 2017).

9 S.K. Sangha, "Valuing Canadian Female Soldiers in the Canadian Armed Forces," NATO Association of Canada, September 8, 2015, http://natoassociation.ca/valuing-canadian-female-soldiers-in-the-canadian-armed-forces/.

10 "Canada's First Female Infantry Officer Opens Up about Harassment, Abuse and Enabling in the Military," *CBC Radio,* March 29, 2018, http://www.cbc.ca/radio/outintheopen/enablers-1.4579817/canada-s-first-female-infantry-officer-opens-up-about-harassment-abuse-and-enabling-in-the-military-1.4580237; N. Mercier and A. Castonguay, "Our Military's Disgrace," *Maclean's,* May 16, 2014, http://www.macleans.ca/news/canada/our-militarys-disgrace/.

11 D. Coates, "The Best Soldiers of All: Unsung Heroines in Canadian Women's Great War Fictions," *Canadian Literature* 151 (1996): 82.

12 Ibid., 84.

13 T.T. Aoki, "In the Midst of Double Imaginaries: The Pacific Community as Diversity and as Difference," *Contents: Pacific Asian Education* 7, 1/2 (1995): 6.

14 Meyer, "Living Inquiry," 86.

15 Matt. 24:6 (Revised Standard Version).

16 Malaal, "Like a Desert Flower," 29.

17 From the monologue "All the world's a stage" in *As You Like It:* B. Mowat, P. Werstine, M. Poston, R. Niles, eds., *As You Like It* (Washington, DC: Folger Shakespeare Library, n.d.), II.vii.73, http://www.folgerdigitaltexts.org.

18 Empress Marie Louise travelled to Blois for refuge in 1814, signalling Napoleon's abdication. M.L. Bonaparte and F. Masson, *The Private Diaries of the Empress Marie-Louise, Wife of Napoleon I* (1814; repr., New York: Appleton & Co., 1922).

19 From Blois in 1429, Joan of Arc prepared to lead the siege of Orléans. From Blois, she also sent her authoritative first letter to the English commander. K. Harrison, *Joan of Arc: A Life Transfigured* (New York: Anchor Books/Penguin, 2014); A. Williamson, *Joan of Arc's First Letter to the English Commanders at Orleans (22 March 1429),* trans. A. Williamson, http://archive.joan-of arc.org/joanofarc_letter_Mar1429.html.

16

Soldiers Lead the Way in the Fight for Mental Health among Men

John S. Ogrodniczuk

OUR SOLDIERS HOLD A special place in my heart. When I think of them, a number comes to mind: 64909. That number was permanently inscribed on my paternal grandfather's arm when he was imprisoned in Auschwitz. My grandfather survived because of the sacrifice of our soldiers.

Now, as then, our soldiers risk their lives for the safety and freedom of others. When they come back from their tours of duty, they often bring back injuries, not all of which we can see. *Contact!Unload* is about working to heal those invisible injuries – the types of injuries that often can have the most profound impact on a person's life.

The play does more than share the courageous journey of soldiers who reveal their wounds and invite others to partake in their healing, as powerful as that story is on its own; it also shows the way for others in our society who may suffer from similar injuries, like depression and anxiety. The significance of having soldiers pave the way for others, especially other men, cannot be overstated. Too often we hear about why so many men don't tackle health challenges like depression or anxiety for such reasons as:

- Men need to be self-reliant.
- Men don't talk about their feelings.
- Men don't show vulnerabilities.
- Men need to be strong.
- Men are supposed to tough it out.

Contact!Unload shows how the toughest men of all – soldiers – break through such stereotypes to tackle their health problems head-on. If these men, who epitomize strength, integrity, selflessness, and courage, are willing to open themselves up and tackle tough health problems like depression and anxiety, then there is no excuse for other men who have similar challenges not to do the same. *Contact!Unload* and the strong men who bring this play to life help normalize health issues like depression and show that they can be overcome.

The play is one of many initiatives at the University of British Columbia that have been developed to bring awareness and respond to the mental health needs of men.[1] Such work attempts to disrupt how men think about mental health and break down the stigma that surrounds the topic. Rather than having men who live with mental illness think they're weak, flawed, or different from other guys, this work helps men recognize that we all occasionally have our struggles and that something like depression, for instance, is fairly common among men. Depression is not a consequence of personal failure – sometimes our coping strategies just get overwhelmed.

This work also tries to shift men's perspectives about health services. Because of the way men tend to be socialized – that is, taught to be men – we often view asking for help (in any form) as something we just don't do. Help seeking is often construed as a sign of weakness that a lot of men want to avoid at all costs.[2] In fact, lots of men will suffer in silence because they can't bring themselves to reach out for a hand. Unfortunately, for too many of them, the consequences can be terrible – men's suicide rates are about four times higher than those of women.[3]

Critical to this effort is the reframing of help seeking as a show of strength, of taking control of one's situation to get things back on track. Reaching out for a hand to get some professional guidance or advice is all about the man grabbing the bull by the horns and saying, "I need to fix some stuff" ("stuff" being a euphemism for something amiss).

In general, men seem reluctant to advocate for their mental health needs, often because they are poorly informed about them.[4] It's time for Canadian men and women to make their voices heard and put their words into action, just like the brave men in *Contact!Unload*. Each of us has a role to play in helping improve the mental health of all members of our society. My role is inspired by Auschwitz prisoner 64909, the selfless soldiers who liberated him and others from the horrid death camps, and the generations of soldiers who followed and continue to serve their country and fellow citizens. Collectively, we need to ask ourselves what we can do to serve them.

Notes
1 J.S. Ogrodniczuk, J.L. Oliffe, D. Kuhl, and P. Gross, "Men's Mental Health: Spaces and Places That Work for Men," *Canadian Family Physician* 62 (2016): 463–64.
2 C.A. Sierra Hernandez, C. Han, J.L. Oliffe, and J.S. Ogrodniczuk, "Understanding Help-Seeking among Depressed Men," *Psychology of Men and Masculinity* 15 (2014): 346–54.

3 J.S. Ogrodniczuk and J.L. Oliffe, "Men and Depression," *Canadian Family Physician* 57 (2011): 153–55.

4 J.S. Ogrodniczuk, J.L. Oliffe, and N. Black, "Canadian Men's Perspectives of Depression: Awareness and Intention to Seek Help," *American Journal of Men's Health* 11 (2017): 877–79.

17

Audience Experience of Vicarious Witnessing in Performing War

Marion Porath, Marla Buchanan, and Elizabeth Banister

> *I sit in anticipation in a small, intimate performance space. I have witnessed*
> Contact!Unload *before but this time, in London, we are much closer to the*
> *performers and the performance for the first time. A vivid tile mural faces us,*
> *its images and text powerful reminders of the tragic impact of war.*[1] *Suddenly a*
> *battle cry pierces the room. Soldiers carry in and erect a Tribute Pole. Names of*
> *soldiers are etched in the wooden coffins that form the pole, agony and despair*
> *portrayed in the rendering of a tattooed soldier. Soldiers and artists crafted the*
> *pole and the mural. The stories and histories represented in these pieces stir my*
> *feelings.*[2] *I am both moved and apprehensive; emotions begin to overwhelm*
> *me. I tell myself to breathe, focus, and appreciate the power and sensitivity. My*
> *intellectual mind knows how the arts bring aesthetics, discipline, and imagina-*
> *tion to understanding complexity*[3] *and how they evoke empathy and under-*
> *standing.*[4] *I know that before me is a repertoire of tools that are "inherently*
> *transdisciplinary,"*[5] *tools that will provoke thinking through their multiple ways*
> *to access and deepen understanding. But my emotional mind is overwhelmed.*
> *The play begins.*
>
> – MARION

PERFORMING WAR IS THE process of conveying the impact of war on the participants to an audience in a theatrical setting. The performance of war has been shown to have significant effects, both positive and negative, on theatre audiences.[6] This chapter features audience responses in the form of intimate narrative accounts of participation as outsiders with insider knowledge to the experience of vicariously witnessing *Contact!Unload.*

The foundation of this chapter considers how the witnessing process affects the self, combining "elements of testimony and reflexivity"[7] of the authors, who have witnessed an average of eight performances. Visual images are part of the narrative, as well as a conversation among the authors about their perspectives of witnessing performativity.

We offer our written reflections to illustrate our shared meaning and learning as witnesses to the creative processes. Through reflection and writing, we came to understand the multiple layers of what it means to serve in the military and how this was embedded in artistic works.[8] Carolyn Wake notes that "spectators function in the moment while operating as witnesses in and through time – as such, bearing witness to trauma injury in performance is an act of temporal delay."[9]

"Because the arts open up the ... audience to emotional moments, feelings enter into the work; the arts ... tap into the cognitive and emotional."[10] "Images that have emotional overtones stay with us ... only to return and provoke at a later time."[11] *Contact!Unload* connected our spectatorial "sensibilities through visceral engagement ... through expressive physicality."[12] Our own "embodied aspect of vision ... drew us into an ambivalent position as viewer of the visual representation of suffering."[13]

Photographs and collaged images augment the narratives of our experiences, highlighting key moments that illuminate our experiences of the play. Like the play that we witnessed that uses performance art to build understanding, visual images provide "new ways with which to perceive and interpret ... ways that make vivid realities that would otherwise go unknown.[14] The use of "artistic modes of representation allows for participation in a different way and may increase the likelihood of making an impact ... on the audience."[15]

The deep personal understanding of the impact of the play upon audience members is presented through the lens of vicarious witnessing. "Vicarious witnessing" is a term that emerged from studies in traumatic stress and is defined as "a process that takes place when a witnessing participant listens to, reads, or observes a narrative or visual representation of a trauma event that a survivor recounts. Vicarious witnessing happens when a person experiences an event through the unique interpretation or perspective of the storyteller or narrator."[16] Patrice Keats explains that vicarious witnessing is a complex process of empathizing with the pain of another. She states that through vicarious witnessing, we are constructing an internal witnessing account, the idea of the "witnessing after-image" that holds on to us.[17] In our vicarious witnessing experience, it becomes evident how the act of witnessing the veterans' performances of their trauma narratives had effects upon us. The closeness to the performance of trauma can "undermine the audience's ability to keep a reflective and emotional distance." In particular, empathy for the performers at the visceral level engages a "transmission of affects that bypasses an intellectual engagement with the performance."[18]

MARION: The impact is profound. Verbal, embodied, visual, and aural portrayals assail me. There is such strength, such profound sensitivity, in the band of brothers performing war. Unity, honour, determination, commitment. My heart aches; my head fails me. After, as I listen to audience members recounting their impressions, I know my words won't come yet but "I like to think that among the forgotten things are treasures, which unexpectedly come back."[19]

Now as I write this (seven months after the performance) much has come back – through thought, talk, and image creation. As they are for the soldiers, images are, for me, a "form of disclosure" of lived reality.[20] The performance shone a light on the military experience – the strong dedication to community, the strength, the deep intelligence and sensitivity brought to the experience, the wounds, the desperate struggles to heal, the commitment to telling the story in ways that allow deeper understanding of what it means to go to war and what it means to come back. No one from my immediate family has gone to war. I knew so little. I can never fully understand the depth of these soldiers' realities; but their images and their performance have given me a richer understanding and appreciation of "what it is like to be at that place."[21] They shone lights on the depth and complexity of what it means to be a soldier.

The evocative cry that began the performance brought back memories of seeing the haka performed. Originally a Maori war dance, the haka is now performed by many citizens of New Zealand, including the military.[22] The movements and loud chants of the haka convey identity, determination, skill, and commitment.[23] Over time, the haka has come to stand for community and strength. It conveys respect, welcome, farewell, challenge, sorrow, happiness, and appreciation. Now I begin to understand how all of these symbolic facets of movement and chant in *Contact!Unload* affected me deeply.

Soldiers can be broken by war but many are strong in the broken places[24] or have a latent strength that is nurtured through repair. Like the Japanese art of *kintsugi* (golden joinery), in which broken ceramic pots are mended with gold, "breaks have a philosophically-rich merit of their own."[25] Something artful, beautiful, and strong can be created in the breaks. *Contact!Unload* conveys the strength of soldiers whose hearts and minds are joined with gold.

Karen Malpede describes theatrical performances as "a theatre of witness."[26] Witnessing a theatrical event based on real-life events requires the audience to

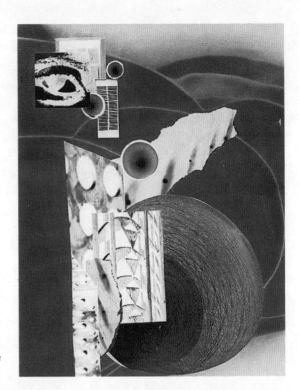

Figure 22 Illuminating the military experience | Collage by Marion Porath.

hold in their imagination the events that transpired. Malpede states that witnessing a traumatic performance allows the audience, and in this case, performers, an opportunity to "reverse trauma's debilitating effects on self and society by giving shape to the complex and cyclical stages of remembrance and recovery."[27]

> MARLA: Watching the play had many emotional impacts on me at various locations over seven viewings. I cried at every one of them but at different points in the play. I cried when Tim[28] said he lost his soul; I cried when Stephen said that his brother's suicide was a choice; I cried when Chuck[29] said that he missed the action in that he would never have that kind of experience again in his life, and when Chuck remembered the soles of the dead soldier's boots; I cried when Warren told the story about the hockey jersey for the boy of the fallen father. I tear up now as I remember these moments in the play. The content of these moments is very moving but I also cry because of my relationship to the veterans sharing these moments.

As a clinician for the Veterans Transition Program (VTP), I know the costs and the price they have personally paid, and so I cry now as an audience member because as a professional I could not cry then.

For me as a woman, the play's strong masculinity felt like a physical assault. The shouting, the physicality of movement, the military language and acronyms displaced me from my inner clinical knowledge. The inner workings of military culture are alien to me, only known to me through the media and my work with the VTP. As a woman it alienates me on gender lines as well. To gain admission to the inner circle, inner language, you need to gain their trust and respect – but how? I struggled to figure out how I would gain entry. How would I be able to assure them that I could "take it" – that I wouldn't fall apart as I witnessed their trauma? So, I armoured myself psychologically and I did not cry. The play allowed me to remove this armour and be present to the pain as myself, a woman whose heart breaks for the price our veterans and their families have to pay.

ELIZABETH: During the past year I have seen four productions of *Contact!-Unload* – two in Vancouver and two in London. Each performance has left me with profound unease and discomfort related to my "own embodiment as a performance presence"[30] in seeing the depth of performers' shared pain of loss, grief, and experience of alienation with the "returning home" process. I was witnessing, first hand, the effects of "the way in which trauma can tear the fabric of peoples' lives without reason or warning."[31] I was "called upon to recognize that there is a relationship between what is shown in the theatre and [my] own experience of the world."[32]

I find it difficult to articulate my experience of viscerally connecting to the performers' physical presence and action. With each performance I was mesmerized; I was drawn into the moment, suspending my sense of time. At the beginning of each performance, I was aware of a stillness that engulfed the intimate, theatrical space created through shortened physical distance between the actors and audience members. Suddenly, loud shouting and marching that came from the stage ripped through my body. I gasped! The visual, auditory, and sensory effects of the play sank painfully and deeply into me. I was not alone. I felt a heightened, palpable shared tension among audience members as we collectively witnessed the action.[33]

Witnessing the play evoked a sense of reverence and deep respect for the men's collective allegiance to the military and to each other.[34] I have been left with a sense of visceral empathy,[35] which has provoked for me many questions: What do the men and the artistic representations of the veteran experience "teach us about ourselves, about the traumatized others, and about the ethics of encounter within performance contexts"?[36] My role as witness promoted a consciousness-raising process of the ethical and political implications of what it means for Canadian men and women to serve. I was confronted with the notion that in my response to the play, I was called to "take responsibility for it."[37] Since observing the play, I have been drawn into an ongoing labour of "observing, interpreting, and reflecting human life"[38] and of questioning the universal and shared meaning of human suffering. What now am I called to do in response to my role as witness to the men's vulnerability?

Attending to Audience Reactions

In addition to the educational and knowledge transfer impacts of this type of performance, as professionals within the fields of counselling psychology and mental health, we recognize that the emotional resonance of the play may be considerable for audience members. Strong reactions and responses to performances such as these are normal and expected. However, audience members may be surprised, taken off guard, or even triggered into distress. In order to prepare audience members and mitigate unexpected reactions, we offer the following recommendations:

1 Inform the audience that the content of the play represents the lived traumatic military experience of soldiers who have served and, as a result, witnesses may experience a range of emotions and physiological responses to the play. In this way, such reactions are normalized. At this time, also remind audience members that people are available to speak with them about their reactions.
2 At the end of the performance, address the audience again with a specific acknowledgment of the emotional impact of the performance. You may even request the audience to check in with themselves and take a few deep breaths together. This signals the end, brings people together, and normalizes what they have experienced.

These preliminary recommendations serve as a starting point and are built on those suggested in the psychological literature as well as the current introductory cautionary and debriefing practices in place at performances of *Contact!Unload*.

As Bessel van der Kolk and other trauma experts explain, having the opportunity to debrief what was witnessed soon after trauma exposure, including vicarious witnessing experiences, is an important self-care strategy and is an ethic of care that needs to be addressed.[39] In terms of performance of war or the theatre of war, there is the potential for transmission of trauma as well as the reliving of one's past trauma experience through this type of exposure. We offer the recommendations above to open up the conversation about performing war within an ethic of care.

Conclusion

The three of us created a group witnessing experience by talking together over tea and sharing breakfasts and dinners together, whenever and wherever we found opportunities, over a two-year period. We shared our responses to aspects of the performance and the artwork, raised questions, and brought our collective experience and new learning to bear on furthering our understanding of performing war. We were drawn to discussing some of the ethics of trauma theatre in which veterans are the live actors. The line between performance and reality is often blurred. We constructed a social understanding of our shared enlistment to the project. For us, the group experience was, and continues to be, a source of deeper understanding and a source of social responsibility. Our experience provides a safe container in which to express our own shock, distress, and worries about the performers, the audience participants, and ourselves.

The group experience helped normalize our experiences of bearing witness to the performers' narratives and helped raise our consciousness of the social and political context within which the storyline took place. Witnessing both the play and other artistic representations invited us to reflect upon our assumptions and attitudes about what it means to devote one's life to one's country. We needed to confront the question: What are we now called to do?

As audience members, we were "a community of individual spectators,"[40] co-creating shared meanings. We talked with the soldiers; we witnessed other audience members' responses during and after performances. Sharing our witness experience was validating in terms of the emotional labour involved in our witnessing role. It also built community – between ourselves, with the soldiers, and with other audience members. Our commitment to attend the performances illustrated our respect for the men. We had a shared understanding of the ethics of supporting the veterans through our active and embodied audience role. We became ambassadors of the work.

Notes

1 An image of the lestweforgetCANADA mural was displayed as audiences entered the performance space. See Chapter 6.

2 T. Whitehead, as cited in R. Howe, ed., *The Quotable Teacher* (Guilford, CT: Lyons Press, 2000).

3 A.L. Cole and J.G. Knowles, "Arts-Informed Research," in *Handbook of the Arts in Qualitative Research,* ed. J.G. Knowles and A.L. Cole, 55–70 (Los Angeles: Sage, 2008).

4 E. Eisner, "Art and Knowledge," in Knowles and Cole, *Handbook of the Arts in Qualitative Research,* 3–12.

5 M. Root-Bernstein and R. Root-Bernstein, "Body Thinking beyond Dance," in *Dance: Current Selected Research,* vol. 5, *Dance Education,* ed. L.Y. Overby and B. Lepczyk (New York: AMS Press, 2005), 194.

6 J. Thompson, J. Hughes, and M. Balfour, *Performance in Place of War* (Calcutta: Seagull Books, 2009).

7 C. Wake, "Book Review: *Theatre of the Real,* by Carol Martin (Basingstoke: Palgrave Macmillan, 2013)," *Performance Paradigm* 11 (2015): 123, http://www.performanceparadigm. net/index.php/journal/article/viewFile/172/169.

8 L. Hassall, "Breaking the Silence: Exploring Experiences of Post-Traumatic Stress Disorder with Returned Veterans to Develop a Contemporary Performance Narrative, *The Return,*" *About Performance* 12 (2014): 27–44.

9 As cited in Hassall, "Breaking the Silence," 41.

10 K.M. Boydell, T. Volpe, S. Cox, A. Katz, et al., "Ethical Challenges in Arts-Based Health Research," *International Journal of the Creative Arts in Interdisciplinary Practice* 11 (2012): 11.

11 Ibid., 10.

12 L. Taylor, "The Experience of Immediacy: Emotion and Enlistment in Fact-Based Theatre," *Studies in Theatre and Performance* 31, 2 (2011): 233.

13 S.A. Oliver, "Trauma, Bodies, and Performance Art: Towards an Embodied Ethics of Seeing," *Continuum* 24, 1 (2010): 128.

14 Eisner, "Art and Knowledge," 11.

15 Boydell et al., "Ethical Challenges in Arts-Based Health Research," 10.

16 P.A. Keats, "Vicariously Witnessing Trauma: Narratives of Meaning and Experience" (PhD dissertation, University of British Columbia, 2003), 11, https://doi.org/10.14288/1.0091215.

17 P.A. Keats, "Vicarious Witnessing in European Concentration Camps: Imagining the Trauma of Another," *Traumatology* 11, 3 (2005): 184.

18 A. de Waal, "Staging Wounded Soldiers: The Affects and Effects of Post-Traumatic Theatre," *Performance Paradigm* 11 (2015): 23, http://performanceparadigm.net/index.php/journal/article/view/170.

19 T. Shinoda, "Works – Bo (Forgotten) in Abstract and Words," *Kateigaho, International Edition* 12 (2006): 17.

20 E. Eisner, "On the Art and Science of Qualitative Research in Psychology," in *Qualitative Research in Psychology: Expanding Perspectives in Methodology and Design,* ed. P.M. Camic, J.E. Rhodes, and L. Yardley (Washington, DC: American Psychological Association, 2003), 24.

21 P.M. Camic, J.E. Rhodes, and L. Yardley, "Naming the Stars: Integrating Qualitative Methods into Psychological Research," in Camic, Rhodes, and Yardley, *Qualitative Research in Psychology,* 10.

22 J. Hutchinson, "New Zealand Soldiers Honour Fallen Comrade with Spine-Tingling Performance of the Haka at Funeral Procession," *Daily Mail,* January 27, 2015, http://www.dailymail.co.uk/news/article-2928238/New-Zealand-Soldiers-honour-fallen-comrade-spine-tingling-performance-haka-funeral-procession.html.

23 Team All Blacks, "The Haka," n.d., http://www.allblacks.com/Teams/Haka.

24 E. Hemingway, *A Farewell to Arms* (New York: Scribner, 1929).

25 The Book of Life, "Kintsugi," 2016, 2, http://www.thebookoflife.org/kintsugi/.
26 K. Malpede, "Chilean Testimonies: An Experiment in Theatre of Witness," *Journal of Contemporary Psychotherapy* 29, 4 (1999): 308.
27 K. Malpede, "Thoughts on a Theatre of Witness and Excerpts from Two Plays of Witness: *Better People, The Beekeeper's Daughter*," in *Genocide, War, and Human Survival*, ed. C.B. Stozier and M. Flynn (Lanham, MD: Rowman and Littlefield, 1996), 233.
28 One of the veterans. See Chapter 11.
29 One of the veterans. See Chapter 2.
30 S.A. Oliver, "Trauma, Bodies, and Performance Art: Towards an Embodied Ethics of Seeing," *Continuum* 24, 1 (2010): 120.
31 P. Duggan, "Feeling Performance, Remembering Trauma," *Platform* 2, 2 (2007): 47.
32 N. Ridout, as cited in P. Duggan, "Others, Spectatorship, and the Ethics of Verbatim Performance," *New Theatre Quarterly* 29, 2 (2013): 155.
33 Duggan, "Feeling Performance, Remembering Trauma."
34 Taylor, "The Experience of Immediacy."
35 Duggan, "Feeling Performance, Remembering Trauma."
36 Taylor, "The Experience of Immediacy," 148.
37 Duggan, "Others, Spectatorship, and the Ethics of Verbatim Performance," 156.
38 J.L. Beck, G. Belliveau, G. Lea, and A. Wager, "Delineating a Spectrum of Research-Based Theatre," *Qualitative Inquiry* 17, 8 (2011): 688.
39 B. van der Kolk, *The Body Keeps the Score: Brain, Mind and Body in the Healing of Trauma* (New York: Viking Books, 2014).
40 Duggan, "Feeling Performance, Remembering Trauma," 54.

18
Understanding the Impacts of
Contact!Unload for Audiences

Jennica Nichols, Susan M. Cox, and George Belliveau

THIS CHAPTER DISCUSSES THE impacts of *Contact!Unload*. We begin by presenting our methods and insights from the Phase III (see Introduction) evaluation of *Contact!Unload* conducted in conjunction with four shows that took place in Vancouver, Ottawa, and Kingston (Canada) in September 2016, along with one filmed viewing in Vancouver in November 2016. Building on this experience, we discuss the design and implementation of the Phase IV evaluation of *Contact!Unload* in September 2017. Within this project, evaluation has been defined as a systematic collection of data to learn about how *Contact!Unload* has impacted the audience. We looked at intended impacts as well as unintended impacts. We conclude by reflecting on evaluation successes as well as lessons learned for research-based theatre, using *Contact!Unload* as our example.

Methods

Phase III Evaluation: Fall 2016
Audience impacts were evaluated using a mixed-methods approach, with data collection immediately following the performance and three to six months after seeing the play to elucidate both immediate and longer-term impacts of *Contact!Unload*.[1] We chose to use a written survey, in-person focus groups, and phone interviews with audience members. The approaches used were informed by evaluation methods used previously in measuring audience experiences of research-based theatre, the expertise of the research team, and available resources.[2]

Post-Performance Quantitative Survey
A written survey was developed with six five-point Likert scale questions:[3]

1 I liked the play.
2 I think the play accurately showed the struggles of veterans returning home from conflict overseas.

3 I think it was essential to the play that the actors were veterans themselves.
4 The play made me more aware of non-physical wounds caused by going to places of conflict.
5 The play made me better understand the need for programs to support the healing of veterans.
6 I think theatre is an effective way to educate Canadians about veterans struggling with mental health in silence.

In addition, the survey contained two demographic questions and space for contact information if the individual wanted to be included in follow-up interviews or focus groups. A hard copy of the survey, included within the play's program, was provided to all audience members as they entered the performance space. An announcement about the survey was included at the start of the show. A clearly identified box on a table was placed near the exit to collect completed surveys, and for one performance, we had a team member designated to collect the survey from audience members. The analysis was conducted in R (Version 3.3.1).[4]

Follow-up Interviews and Focus Groups
We conducted three focus groups and four interviews in February 2017. These were all facilitated by a clinical counsellor (Carson Kivari) who was able to provide therapeutic support if any participant felt triggered during data collection. Of the forty-five audience members who provided contact information in the post-performance survey, eighteen agreed to participate. Focus groups lasted approximately 120 minutes and were hosted over three evenings at a downtown Vancouver location. The four phone interviews lasted thirty to sixty minutes and were arranged for audience members who were unable to attend a focus group.

The same semi-structured guide was used for both interviews and focus groups. The five guiding questions were:

1 What were some of the main messages of the play?
2 Did seeing the play affect your understanding of issues related to veterans?
3 Have you discussed the play with anyone after seeing it?
4 Has anything happened in your life that was influenced by seeing the play?
5 What do you think about using theatre to present this type of work?

All focus groups and interviews were audio-recorded and all participants consented to share their views for research purposes.

George and Jennica listened closely to the audio-recorded interviews and a transcription of relevant sections was undertaken in order to engage in the qualitative analysis. The authors then engaged in a thematic analysis in which they independently looked for patterns in audience responses pertinent to the play's impacts on audience members.[5] Themes and subthemes were compared with any discrepancies discussed until a consensus was reached. In the following paragraphs, we briefly explore the results of our initial evaluation. For a more detailed discussion, see George Belliveau and Jennica Nichols's article "Audience Responses to *Contact!Unload.*"[6]

Demographics

A total of 116 people filled out the survey with 68 percent of the sample being civilians (*n* = 72), 8 percent military (*n* = 8), and 25 percent friends or family of someone in the military (*n* = 26). Of those who participated in the follow-up focus groups and interviews, 78 percent were civilians (*n* = 14), while 11 percent were military personnel (*n* = 2), and 11 percent were connected to someone in the military as a family member or friend (*n* = 2).

Key Themes

Theme 1: Veterans as Performers Is Important to Audience Impacts

All but one actor in the September 2016 iteration of *Contact!Unload* were current or former members of the military. The survey found that 96 percent of respondents (*n* = 110) thought it was important to have veterans depict their own stories. Focus group members emphasized that having real veterans as the performers increased the authenticity for the audience: "You could hear it in their voice, it was real, it was raw ... not acting, not sugar-coated" (Civilian, Focus Group 2). The authenticity of the veteran performers was seen as directly related to emotional and cognitive impacts reported by civilians. For instance, one respondent suggested that the impacts were much deeper because "you know that they've done it, and they tell their own stories" (Civilian, Focus Group 1). Another person commented that because the play used veterans, "it didn't feel like acting when I was watching it. It felt like I was very intimately watching someone experience something that was real. I almost felt like I was intruding on someone's very private moment of healing" (Civilian, Focus Group 1). Having veterans perform in *Contact!Unload* was also seen as important to those in the military. A participant who currently serves as a medic in the Canadian Armed Forces said that "hearing the play from my peers really drove it home" (Military, Interview 2). He went on to talk about how he felt proud to hear these veterans tell their story and bare their souls in front of a public audience.

Several focus group participants highlighted the immense bravery of the veterans to perform their own stories or stories of other veterans in front of an audience: "I felt a huge amount of gratitude to them. That they would actually step up ... and educate us, to bring us into their world a little bit, to come into our world to show it to us. I just, to me that is a lot of courage" (Civilian, Focus Group 1).

Theme 2: Play Raises Awareness and Knowledge of Veterans' Issues

In showing the difficult transition from soldier to civilian life, *Contact!Unload* aimed to raise awareness of the stress and psychological injuries that many of our soldiers bring home as a result of their military service. The play also intended to raise awareness of opportunities for veterans to heal and cope by showing the veterans seeking professional counselling and support from their fellow veterans. Rather than an outside voice reporting on these topics, *Contact!Unload* allows the audience to experience this through first-hand accounts by the veterans.

Eighty-nine percent of survey respondents reported that *Contact!Unload* increased their awareness of non-physical wounds veterans suffer by going to places of conflict ($n = 103$). The focus groups highlighted several ways the play did this. One audience member spoke about

the ways in which the stress and anxiety and trauma can materialize and how it can materialize differently for each person. Some of the characters responded to it by being a little overzealous ... wanting to commit to another tour while for another person it was a lot of anger, and for another person it was kind of being sombre, really keeping to himself, denial. (Family or Friend, Interview 3)

Audience members also discussed a new understanding about what causes trauma for veterans, with one audience member explaining that the play made her realize that "you don't need to be on the frontlines to see something that can be traumatic. Just being there can have an effect on you" (Civilian, Focus Group 3). Another participant noted that anyone could suffer from psychological issues after being in a combat zone, regardless of age, rank, and previous experience, and that it is "probably not a matter of if you're going to be affected but rather when, and at what level, and how" (Military, Interview 2). The play was also seen to have increased awareness of the many different factors that might cause mental health challenges for veterans.

Ninety-six percent of survey respondents agreed that the play increased their understanding of the need for support programs for veterans ($n = 110$). Multiple participants talked about a new understanding of the magnitude of veterans' psychological issues with respect to overall prevalence, "the need for help being quite great among veterans" (Civilian, Focus Group 2). Others felt that the play highlights how veterans' issues remain invisible to the general public as "a lot of people don't know the suffering that goes on" (Civilian, Focus Group 1). In addition, the play seems to have raised people's awareness about how "it was important for those guys [veterans] to find somebody they can talk to" (Civilian, Focus Group 2). One respondent highlighted the play's key message that "it's okay to come out and tell your family and tell your friends about [mental health issues] because that will actually help you" (Civilian, Focus Group 3). Several people became aware that effective support is available for veterans: "It was exciting to me to know there is some therapy that does succeed ... to see something where people had found a way to successfully help these people with the issues" (Civilian, Focus Group 2).

Lastly, many audience members felt the play helped to address current stigma around mental health and seeking help. As one person highlighted, the play was "trying to address the stigma around it [post-traumatic stress] and trying to encourage people to seek help ... to feel comfortable and okay" (Family or Friend, Interview 3). These comments point to how audience members took away new insights, and how the play generated a platform to engage and inform the public on the topic of veterans and some of the post-deployment challenges they face.

Theme 3: Theatre as a Viable Medium for Sharing of Veterans' Experiences

This initial evaluation explored the audience's perspectives on how the medium of theatre might serve to share the stories of veterans and the group therapeutic model of the Veterans Transition Program (VTP). The survey found almost everyone (97 percent) felt that theatre was an appropriate medium for educating people about veterans' mental health struggles. The qualitative analysis also explored what audiences perceived as being unique in the medium of theatre. Some focus group participants spoke about the emotional impacts theatre offered to the veterans' stories: "I've never been to a play where I've felt like this ... it's real life, a unique hybrid of theatre and real life" (Civilian, Focus Group 1). What lingered for several participants was a felt experience that humanized veterans and their struggles, as theatre engaged both the cognitive and the emotional through its liveness. One participant suggests that "putting a human face to the issues makes it vivid. You read about it in the paper or hear it on the radio/TV, but this play made it real. It's humanizing" (Focus Group 3). *Contact!Unload* was also seen as shedding new light on veterans by challenging existing stereotypes: "I had this stereotype of army guys before ... like they just want to go fire guns or something, and that's why you would go, and join the army. But I feel like after watching the play ... that was sort of destroyed for me (Civilian, Focus Group 1).

Another observation made by a few participants was that the medium of theatre creates a forum where audience members witness a shared experience both during and after the performance. This idea was extended by an interview participant who suggested that with theatre, "you get to share it with other people at the same time, so it's not an isolated experience ... you feel connected to a community" (Civilian, Interview 1). The humanity and emotional connection the veterans offered in the production surfaced as an essential component of the audience impacts. This suggests how live theatre may provide a valuable mechanism for informing and educating a public as well as activating a visceral and emotional response to issues veterans face.

Phase IV Evaluation: Fall 2017

The revival of *Contact!Unload* in the fall of 2017 gave us an opportunity to revisit and further our evaluation of the project. There were four areas where we wanted to improve upon our initial evaluation in order to gain a deeper understanding of audience impacts. First, we wanted to add pre-performance questions that would enable us to directly measure changes in awareness and understanding (i.e., not self-reported). Second, we wanted to adapt our data collection methods to better integrate the evaluation activities into the overall theatre event. Third, we sought a larger sample for our post-performance written survey to more thoroughly establish how changes in awareness and understanding of veterans' mental health issues were self-reported. Finally, we wanted to create opportunities for audience members to share their thoughts in an open-ended, qualitative way following the show.

Including a short pre-performance component enabled us to establish a baseline so that we could measure changes in awareness and knowledge related to experiencing *Contact!Unload*. This component included three items asked immediately before and after the performance: 1) there is currently enough help available for veterans; 2) every solider in a conflict zone is at risk of non-physical injuries like post-traumatic stress disorder (PTSD); and 3) I am confident that I understand what someone with PTSD looks like. Respondents used clickers to select responses (in real-time) from a five-point

Likert scale ranging from "strongly disagree" to "strongly agree" to answer each question. A clicker is a battery-run handheld device with five buttons labelled A to E. Questions were asked with possible responses also labelled A to E that were projected onto a screen on the stage and read out loud by the musician (Carson Kivari). Audience members pushed the button with the letter that corresponded to their answer and the value was recorded electronically. We chose to use clickers rather than paper-based surveys in order to integrate pre-performance and post-performance data collection into the overall theatre experience. Completion rates ranged from 84 to 99 percent.

We also added a military-themed art-based installation made of camouflage army net. Audience members were encouraged to write a response to the prompt "One message or idea that I will take away with me from the performance is ..." on a blank paper tag. They were then invited to attach their tag to the artwork. We used different coloured stickers for each performance to link responses with each show. Additional data collection activities included audience observations conducted by two researchers during each of the six September 2017 performances.

An online follow-up survey that included both Likert scale and open-ended questions was distributed six months after the fall 2017 performances. Interested audience members provided their contact information either when they reserved tickets online or at the door before the performance. Of the 180 of people who provided contact information, 81 (45 percent) responded to the survey. We also completed two more follow-up focus groups ($n = 10$) and one phone interview in Vancouver in March 2018, six months after the fall 2017 performances. These focus groups and the interview included the voices of veterans, family members of veterans, and civilians. At the time of writing this chapter, we are in the process of analyzing the results.

Perhaps the most significant difference in our Phase IV evaluation was integration of the evaluation into the overall theatre experience. For example, we had the musician come onstage before the performance and again before the post-performance talkback to guide the audience through the pre-performance and post-performance surveys. This created the space for audience members to do the evaluation during the overall theatre experience. We also reframed the evaluation as an opportunity for the audience to be part of the theatre experience. As one audience member reflected: "The fact that we had the little gadgets [electronic clickers] that we can register, you know, certain questions and feelings ... you just felt like you're interacting, you're part of it. You got us all really involved in the play" (Civilian, Focus Group 5).

Discussion and Implications

The audience feedback gathered from *Contact!Unload* sheds new light on the audience impacts of theatre with veterans. The data collected suggest that using theatre was an effective medium for educating and engaging the public around some of the veterans' issues and the available supports. Through our two evaluations, several lessons were learned about what practices and approaches worked well, and areas of improvement that may be helpful to future research-based theatre projects. We are, of course, conscious that each project is unique; the suggestions here are meant as guides for consideration in order to improve the evaluation of impacts on audience members who watch research-based theatre performances.

Methods to Evaluate Impacts of the Performance on the Audience

It is important to think about measuring impacts of the performance on audience members and various forms of audience engagement at the conceptualization stage of a research-based theatre project so that the intended outcomes can inform both project and audience evaluation designs. Budget, team expertise, and project timelines should also be considered when selecting methods for understanding audience impacts.

Developing Measurement Tools

It is critical to connect the project's expected outcomes with the measurement tool by first explicitly identifying expected outcomes. Our strategy was to have evaluation team members brainstorm possible outcomes (i.e., What would a successful project look like for me? What do I think the audience will take away from watching this play?) and to review findings from other research-based theatre projects. Questions used to structure the interview/focus group guide were developed on the basis of the results of the post-performance survey along with project objectives and team feedback. Our experience reveals that pre- and post-performance measurement tools are most effective when it is possible for participants to complete them relatively quickly (i.e., limit the open-ended questions, use primarily Likert scale or true/false response formats). It is also important to pilot the tool with people outside the project to ensure that the language is accessible and the length of the survey is appropriate.

Lessons for Increasing Audience Participation

In our initial evaluation when utilizing a paper-based survey, we found that having a dedicated person responsible for gathering surveys increased our response rate. This person was able to prompt audience members about the survey by asking them whether they had filled it out, along with answering questions and providing copies of the survey and/or a pen if needed. In our fall 2017 evaluation of audience impacts, we found that integrating data collection activities into the overall theatre experience resulted in even greater audience participation. We therefore recommend that a project member be dedicated to facilitate any data collection activities with the audience and that evaluation procedures be integrated into the theatre experience.

Arts-Based Evaluation

The addition of a military-themed art-based installation in the Phase IV evaluation created an opportunity for audience members to share some of their immediate thoughts using their own words. A total of 173 audience members attached comments to the camouflage net, with participation ranging from 23 to 49 percent of the total audience at each show. It was also a unique way to invite the audience to be part of the event, as all comments remained on the net and were thus available to future audience members to engage with. While the analysis of the comments is ongoing, we wanted to share some to highlight the depth and variety of comments provided by the audience. Many comments expressed gratitude towards the veterans who performed and described how the play impacted the individual, including: "My dad served in WWII ... I understand his wounds better. Thank you" and "This information/knowledge will help me take care of my 30 troops. Thank you very much" (anonymous responses). Several comments focused on the impact of having seen the veterans sharing their stories and emotions openly onstage – for example, "incredibly moving – good to see men share" (anonymous responses). Other comments spoke directly to the veterans, such as, "Your strength to be open is inspirational." Based on the positive audience response to this approach, we encourage others to think about how they can use arts-based evaluation methods to invite and display comments about audience impacts.

Lessons from Follow-up Interviews and Focus Groups

Follow-up activities require a budget to provide tokens of appreciation to participants, including group refreshments, and to pay for staff to facilitate the sessions and analyze the data. We recommend that teams consider follow-up activities at the time of project design. People looking to understand the longer-term impacts of their project need to ensure that they collect contact information from individuals at the performance. We created a space for people to provide their contact information and consent to be contacted for follow-up activities when they signed up for tickets online, and we also offered a paper form for people to sign up at the door. Our follow-up activities occurred six months after the performance, to provide insights on long-term resonances that the theatre piece generated. For our focus groups, we used a neutral, fact-based initial question (What do you think the main messages of the play were?) to enable people to recall the play and ease them into sharing within the group. We encourage others to plan for follow-up activities within their projects to understand longer-term impacts of research-based theatre.

Limitations

This study has some potential limitations. For example, we do not know the exact number of audience members who attended the shows in our initial 2016 evaluation as all shows were free and most were without tickets. It is therefore impossible to determine response rates for the written post-performance survey in the initial evaluation. We would therefore encourage future projects to designate a team member to count audience members during each performance, so an accurate response rate can be calculated. Moreover, people self-selected to fill out our surveys. It is unclear whether there was response bias, where those who responded differed from those who did not respond to the survey. We believe that integrating the evaluation into the overall performance helped to minimize this potential bias in our Phase IV evaluation as a much higher proportion of the audience participated in the evaluation. Another limitation is the possibility of self-selection involving those who choose to attend our performances and who therefore may be different from a general audience (e.g., they may be more familiar with theatre and/or veterans' issues compared with the general public). That said, this is almost always the case with research-based theatre unless the performance is part of a research study where audience members are deliberately recruited based on explicit inclusion criteria. Lastly, the responses were very positive. This lack of negative responses to the play may have been due to appreciation for a new awareness of issues that outweighed a critical focus, first-hand knowledge of the project team or those in the play, and/or the felt experience's trumping of more cognitive critiques.

Final Thoughts

While additional resources are required, we believe that evaluating the impacts of research-based theatre on the audience is an essential step in discovering whether a project is meeting its intended objectives. That is, are audience members learning and remembering the intended key messages of the play? By generating a space for formal feedback, projects are better informed about how their intended messages are being received by audiences; this information is helpful for funders, policy makers, and stakeholders. As the methodology continues to evolve, it is essential to adapt evaluation to fit into the theatre space in order to capture the breadth and depth of audience impacts. The evaluation should strive to add value to the overall project.

Research-based theatre is an interdisciplinary approach that offers unique opportunities for knowledge generation and knowledge mobilization. The Phase IV evaluation has made us even more hopeful about the varied and far-reaching impacts research-based theatre can have on audience members. For example, a veteran from the audience shared the following during a focus group:

Even though I have been in the army now for 18 years, this year was the first time I ever spoke at a Remembrance Day ceremony ... I think that, that did have something to do with me seeing *Contact!Unload* actually. I felt like I should become more involved because we don't have enough advocacy for veterans in general. (Veteran, Focus Group 5)

In the same focus group, a family member told us, "I would say the play [made a difference by] being the catalyst for him [husband who is a veteran] getting more personal help" (Family or Friend, Focus Group 5).

The evaluation process has also alerted us to the need to recognize lateral forms of violence arising from the veterans' experiences of trauma that affect those around them. For example, a civilian respondent bravely shared the following information about her response to *Contact!Unload* in an unsolicited email in response to the follow-up online survey:

In my early 20s, I was engaged to a member of the [branch of Canadian military] ... our relationship had been fairly healthy. However, about one year into his active duty, he raped me ... Watching *Contact!Unload* provided me with a little more insight into why he may have done what he did. I'm not saying that it was right or okay, but seeing the anger in the men during the performance made me realize that perhaps he had experienced something traumatic.[7]

This heartfelt testimony speaks to the ripple effect of unaddressed trauma where family members and friends are deeply affected. There is a need to be aware of this residual effect in order to better support veterans transitioning to civilian life. It also highlights a silence within *Contact!Unload* and points to the need to address issues of gender in productions about veterans, mental health, and trauma. The lack of female and racialized voices in the performance was also identified in other evaluation responses.

These two examples emphasize the diversity of experiences with trauma and transitioning back to civilian life that future iterations of this work should consider. *Contact!Unload* was initially conceived and funded by a men's mental health initiative (Movember Canada), and thus had a focus on men's health and men's stories. The evaluation enabled us to learn about how *Contact!Unload* impacted audiences, including identifying important gaps that future interventions need to address in order to continue existing (and foster new) discussions about how we can better support veterans transitioning back to civilian life.

Acknowledgments
Special thank you to Marv Westwood, Foster Eastman, Carson Kivari, Graham Lea, Liam Peel, and Chris Cook for helping with our evaluations.

Notes
This chapter is derived in part from an article published in *Cogent Arts and Humanities* by George Belliveau and Jennica Nichols, July 8, 2017, © 2017 The Authors under a Creative Commons Attribution (CC-BY) 4.0 licence (http://creativecommons.org/licenses/by/4.0/), available online: https://doi.org/10.1080/23311983.2017.1351704.

1 This research was approved by the University of British Columbia Behavioural Research Ethics Board #H15-00111.

2 To date, it is uncommon in research-based theatre to include pre-performance assessments to evaluate the show's impacts on the audience.

3 A Likert scale is used to measure a person's opinions, attitudes, and perceptions. Rather than asking whether the person has experienced (e.g,. yes or no) or believes (e.g., agree or disagree) something, a Likert scale measures how *strongly* they experience or believe it. In our work, our scale had five levels: strongly disagree, somewhat disagree, neither agree or disagree, somewhat agree, and strongly agree.

4 R Development Core Team, *R: A Language and Environment for Statistical Computing* (version 3.3.1) (Vienna: R Foundation for Statistical Computing, 2016), http://www.R-project.org.

5 V. Braun and V. Clarke, "Using Thematic Analysis in Psychology," *Qualitative Research in Psychology* 3, 2 (2006): 77–101; J. Saldaña, *The Coding Manual for Qualitative Researchers* (Thousand Oaks, CA: Sage, 2015).

6 G. Belliveau and J. Nichols, "Audience Responses to *Contact!Unload*: A Canadian Research-Based Play about Returning Military Veterans," *Cogent Arts and Humanities* 4, 1 (2017): 1351704, https://doi.org/10.1080/23311983.2017.1351704.

7 Written consent was obtained to use an anonymous version of the letter as part of the evaluation data.

19

Vulnerable Strength Seen

JS Valdez and Jennica Nichols

JENNICA: This chapter is focused on Phase IV[1] of *Contact!Unload,* which took place in Vancouver and Toronto in September 2017. It explores an interactive installation that was one aspect of the overall evaluation to assess audience impacts of seeing the play. It consisted of a camouflage net and, at some shows, images of artwork created by veterans and artist Foster Eastman.[2] At the end of each performance, audience members were invited to contribute to this installation by writing a response to the prompt, "One message or idea that I will take away with me from the performance is ..." They would write their thoughts on a white card, then tie their message to the camouflage net. A total of 174 audience members participated across six performances.

The interactive installation was the only opportunity for audience members to anonymously provide qualitative feedback immediately after witnessing the play and post-performance talkback. Several people came up to me to express their appreciation for the opportunity to "speak back" to the performers. A number of audience members wrote directly to the performers (e.g., "You are not alone," "Courage takes many forms. You help us see this"). Twenty-seven of the comments (15 percent) included "thanks" or "thank you" towards the veterans for their service and/or for their courage to be onstage. Some audience members spoke about a new awareness or knowledge (e.g., "Some of the hardest battles are fought when veterans come back"), while others shared a personal impact of watching the show (e.g., "I feel fear turn to hope") or general praise for the play (e.g., "Thanks so much for all Canadians. Fantastic play").

As I read JS Valdez's poem "Vulnerable Strength Seen" (below), I am surprised by how many of my thoughts and feelings about being part of *Contact!Unload* are reflected. I feel a resurgence of my own gratitude towards the veterans for sharing their stories and giving me a new understanding of words like service, brotherhood, and sacrifice. I feel that familiar frustration at the lack of diversity onstage (e.g., women and people of colour) and my longing to hear these stories. I am made aware of how my thinking has expanded about the challenges and opportunities faced by veterans when they transition back to civilian life. I also realize how *Contact!Unload* has transformed the concepts of veterans and an operational stress injury from the abstract to something quite real for me. This poem reminds me how much strength it takes to share your vulnerabilities, and that, through this brave sharing, comes both personal growth and deeper connection (or "it takes a lot of strength to unfuck your shit"[3] as the play aptly puts it).

The installation, and its interpretation through this poem, allow us to study audience impacts of *Contact!Unload* in novel ways.[4] For example, the interactive installation has helped us have a more nuanced understanding of audience impacts by letting audience members describe it in their own words. My personal experience with the installation and reading JS Valdez's poem makes my inner evaluator jump with excitement over the future possibilities around art-based evaluation to assess research-based theatre.

The following found poem[5] written by JS Valdez was created from the 174 audience responses.

Vulnerable Strength Seen
a poem by JS Valdez

War real
Real powerful performance
See men share
Wounds heal
Everyone is wounded.
Include female

Real war
Don't suffer in silence
Start Talking
Someone talking with men
Connections made, the audience
They're feeling, for all Canadians
All Canadians feeling
War real

Hope takes strength
Strength takes support
Group sharing needed
Play life.

Peace takes courage
People sharing stories
Share courage.
Play life.

They are one in darkness
Carry on. I will try too.
To be. I am
The beauty of touch.
You and I
Hardest battles are fought
When it's okay to ask for help

PTSD is invisible
You can't just duck
many cases
invisible alone
174 tears

Hope takes strength
Strength takes support
Group sharing needed
Play life.

Peace takes courage
People sharing stories
Share courage.
Play life.

Thank you,

amazing
inspiring
veterans.

JS VALDEZ: As a female artist-researcher involved in the original ensemble that devised and produced *Contact!Unload*, my interpretations are informed by my gendered perspective. When composing the poem, I used a process of word selection that relied largely on numbers rather than personal filters. By numbers I mean using software to create a word cloud, which was one layer of my creative writing process. I used Word Cloud Add-On, a Google Docs add-on, which counted the frequency of each word as they appear in the data.[6] Based on that word count, the software made an image of the most frequently occurring words. The most frequently used words were the largest in the cloud. Based on the largest words (indicating those found most often in the data), I composed repeating stanzas to emphasize the sentiments voiced by many participants. In addition to the analysis of the data with Google Docs to generate the word cloud, I added an additional artistic layer of analysis to the image of words in composing the repeating stanzas. The stanzas that do not repeat were "found" from within the raw data. I took creative licence with word order but did not add or adjust any text that did not exist in the raw data.

Found poetry is a form of poetry in which "words found in a non-poetic context" (in this case, audience responses from the interactive installation) are arranged "into lines that convey a verse rhythm."[7] By this process, data are synthesized by the writing process and represented in a new poetic form. Elizabeth Meyer identifies several educational researchers who have shown found poetry to be a "valuable approach for analysis and representation."[8] Because my found poem distills writings made by participants, it may be thought of as a collaboration between audiences (also research participants) and myself (the poet).

It is indeed a courageous act of generosity to share a story of trauma – courageous in the sense of exposing a vulnerable heart, in the process of which generosity is bestowed upon others. The same may be said of the audiences who witnessed the play. An audience is made vulnerable by having emotional responses elicited by the performances, and those who contributed to the evaluations were most generous not only with their time and attention in watching the play but also in adding their personal written responses. Thank you to the veterans who gave life to *Contact!Unload* so that others might reconsider theirs. And thank you to the audiences who made available their minds and hearts to connect with the veterans.

Notes

1 See Introduction.
2 The artwork was part of Eastman's SERIOUSshit project. See Chapter 6 in this volume.
3 See Moment 21 in the Annotated Playscript in this volume.
4 See Chapter 18.
5 Merriam-Webster, "Found Poem," https://www.merriam-webster.com/dictionary/found%20poem.
6 See http://learnin60seconds.com.
7 Merriam-Webster, "Found Poem."
8 E.J. Meyer, "'Who We Are Matters': Exploring Teacher Identity through Found Poetry," *Learning Landscapes* 2, 1 (2008): 196, http://www.learninglandscapes.ca/index.php/learnland/article/view/Who-We-Are-Matters-Exploring-teacher-Identities-Through-Found-Poetry.

Conclusion

George Belliveau and Graham W. Lea

THIS COMMUNITY- AND university-based project with military veterans has had considerable reach. Over eighty people have been part of the creative and organizational team, and by end of 2019, over 3,500 audience members have witnessed the production. The contributors to this book represent only a small portion of those who have experienced the work. Nonetheless, they bring richly diverse perspectives to their experiences and agree that the conversations raised through *Contact!Unload* are vital. The Veterans Transition Program (VTP) and similar programs are of life-and-death importance to veterans and to their places within their families and the broader social fabric. To be impactful, these programs need to be well supported, but, equally important, veterans and their families need to know they exist and of their potential for positive transformative change. The significant outreach of *Contact!Unload* created a space for veterans and families to learn about the VTP and the possibilities it provides for helping to transition to civilian life while living with stress injuries.

As all citizens are participants in their government's decisions to send soldiers into combat, they are also responsible for understanding the struggles and lasting impacts on soldiers and for advocating for veteran transition supports. Arts productions such as *Contact!Unload* are one way of helping extend the reach of these voices and stories. This sharing can be transformative for both performers and audiences. The production of *Contact!Unload* incorporated community-produced visual art and theatre for both healing and communication on the part of the veterans, and deep, emotional, and transformative witnessing on the part of veteran and non-veteran participants and audiences. While the potential audience of a research-based theatre production such as *Contact!Unload* is limited due to the practicalities of theatre production, drawing together the script and responses to the work in this book helps to extend the learning and outreach of the project.

Through its polyphonic voices, we hope this book offers insights on how an arts-based research process can humanize the challenging experience of returning veterans. The performance brought to life an issue of utmost importance – veterans' successful transition to civilian life post-deployment. As a university/community collaboration, this project exemplifies university research that reaches out to the community and performs a deeply important social service while maintaining academic and aesthetic integrity. Each of the contributors to this book shares a unique piece of the *Contact!Unload* story through participation in or witnessing of the performance. Together, they continue to explore what it means to, and how do we ever, come home, fully.

Contributors

Michael Balfour is a professor of theatre and performance at the University of New South Wales in Sydney, Australia. He is a theatre researcher and practitioner and has written widely on the social and creative applications of theatre, with a particular interest in theatre in conflict and peace building, prison theatre, theatre and migration, theatre in mental health with returning military personnel, and most recently, creative aging and dementia. His most recent books include *Applied Theatre: Understanding Change* (Springer, 2018); and *Performing Arts in Prisons* (Intellect, 2019).

Elizabeth Banister is a professor emerita of nursing at the University of Victoria and is a registered nurse and registered psychologist. She has a private psychology practice in Victoria that includes working with veterans and their families.

George Belliveau is a professor of theatre/drama education at the University of British Columbia. His research interests include research-based theatre, drama and social justice, drama and L2 learning, drama across the curriculum, drama and health research, and Canadian theatre. His scholarly and creative writing can be found in various arts-based and theatre education journals, along with chapters in edited books. He has written or edited six books, including one co-edited with Graham Lea, *Research-Based Theatre: An Artistic Methodology* (Intellect, 2016).

Marla Buchanan is a professor of counselling psychology in the Department of Educational and Counselling Psychology, and Special Education at the University of British Columbia. Her research and clinical practice involve work with various populations exposed to traumatic events, including members of the military, refugees, women in prisons, and people affected by childhood trauma.

Christopher Cook recently completed his MA in counselling psychology at the University of British Columbia. With a background as an actor and a playwright, Chris is passionate about utilizing theatre as a therapeutic, learning, and research tool. His plays include *Quick Bright Things* (Persephone Theatre, 2017) and *Voices UP!* (UBC Learning Exchange, 2017), a collaborative creation with community members in Vancouver's Downtown Eastside.

Susan M. Cox is an associate professor in the W. Maurice Young Centre for Applied Ethics and the School of Population and Public Health at the University of British Columbia. Her research interests include narratives of health and illness, experiences of participants in health research, and ethical and other implications of using the arts as a form of inquiry, as well as knowledge translation. Her scholarly and creative work is published in arts-based and qualitative research journals, along with chapters in edited books.

Britney Dennison is deputy director of the Global Reporting Centre at the University of British Columbia. She is also a producer for the Global Reporting Program. Her work at the GRC has won numerous awards, including several Edward R. Murrow awards, an Online Journalism award, and a Canadian Association of Journalists award. Her work has appeared in the *Toronto Star, The Tyee,* NBC News, CTV, and Al Jazeera.

Heather Duff, a poet and playwright, holds a PhD in drama education from the University of British Columbia. Her poetry and fiction have been published in numerous literary journals and anthologies, and she was a finalist for *The Malahat Review*'s 2011 Long Poem Prize. Heather is the artistic director of Vancouver Youth Theatre, where she directs collaborative, issue-based plays. She is also an instructor in Continuing Studies at Simon Fraser University. Heather was an audience member for the premiere of *Contact!Unload* at Studio 1398, in April 2015, and at a remounting of the play at the Seaforth Armoury, Vancouver, September 2017.

Foster Eastman is a multimedia artist whose work examines social and cultural issues often shrouded in taboo and stigma. Recent exhibits have considered diverse issues, including the atrocities that occurred in China under Mao Zedong and the challenges returning veterans from Afghanistan face as they reintegrate into civilian life. His most recent works collaborating with soldiers were showcased on Parliament Hill, in the Canadian War Museum, and at

Canada House in London, attended by Prince Harry and Prince Charles. Along with the current SERIOUSshit project, these installations were included in the cultural programming and showcased at the 2017 Invictus Games in Toronto.

Lynn Fels is a professor of arts education at Simon Fraser University, where she focuses on drama education, arts for social change, learning through the arts, arts-based research, writing as inquiry, and performative inquiry. Lynn co-edited with Ruth Elwood Martin, Mo Korchinski, and Carl Leggo *Arresting Hope* (2014) and *Releasing Hope* (2019), collections of writings by women with incarceration experience, about their challenges, frustrations, and hopes both within and beyond prison gates. She was an audience member for the June 16, 2016, reading of *Contact!Unload,* attended a rehearsal and performance of *Contact!Unload* in April 2015, and was a participant of the symposium on *Contact!Unload* held at the University of British Columbia in June 2016.

Timothy Garthside is a veteran of Afghanistan and deployed on Operation Archer in January 2006. Tim is currently a student at the University of Victoria, pursuing his undergraduate degree in social work with his sights set on becoming a therapist. He participated in most versions of *Contact!Unload,* portraying himself.

Alistair G. Gordon holds an MA in counselling psychology from the University of British Columbia. He is a registered clinical counsellor in private practice, director of Wellspring Counselling in Vancouver (wellspringcounselling. ca), a counsellor with the BC Public Service, and an adjunct professor in the Department of Counselling Psychology at UBC. Alistair may be contacted at alistair.gordon@alumni.ubc.ca.

Anna Keefe holds a PhD in Language and Literacy Education from the University of British Columbia and continues her research and action in the areas of collaborative program design, arts education, and trauma-informed practice. She supported the development and production of *Contact!Unload* at Granville Island in April/May 2015 as an assistant and witness.

Carson A. Kivari, MA, RCC, is owner and operator of Thrive Downtown Counselling Centre. His counselling space serves individuals, couples, groups, and graduate students within the community. When not directing Thrive, Carson provides trauma-focused counselling for military veterans as well as clinical training for group facilitators as part of his work with the Veterans Transition Network. Carson is also a long-time recording artist, filmmaker, and creative educator.

Tim Laidler is a veteran of the conflict in Afghanistan. He holds an MA in counselling psychology from the University of British Columbia. He is currently the executive director of the UBC Faculty of Education's Centre for Group Counselling and Trauma and a founder and president of the Veterans Transition Network.

Graham W. Lea is an assistant professor of theatre/drama education at the University of Manitoba. His research interests include research-based theatre methodology, narrative in mathematics education, and theatre/drama in health and teacher education research. Graham speaks and publishes widely on theatre education and research methodology. He has been involved in theatre for twenty-five years, working variously as a playwright, stage manager, director, actor, musician, and technician. He is co-editor, with George Belliveau, of the book *Research-Based Theatre: An Artistic Methodology* (Intellect, 2016).

Carl Leggo was a poet and professor in the Department of Language and Literacy Education at the University of British Columbia. He was an audience member for the theatrical performance of *Contact!Unload* at Studio 1398 on Granville Island in May 2015. Sadly, Dr. Leggo passed away during the writing of this book.

Phillip Lopresti is currently a lieutenant in the Canadian Armed Forces and is a member of the Seaforth Highlanders of Canada. He was a civilian when he joined the *Contact!Unload* project as an actor. As a student pursuing a master's degree in counselling psychology during the project, he looked at literature about the arts and storytelling, and how these modalities can enable psychological healing for post-traumatic stress.

Chuck MacKinnon, CD, RT, is a veteran of peacekeeping and Afghanistan. He currently serves as a lieutenant-colonel and commanding officer of the Royal Westminster Regiment and is employed with Canada Post. He participated in all productions of *Contact!Unload* and continues to provide assistance to Dr. Marv Westwood and the University of British Columbia as a military adviser.

Candace Marshall is a PhD student in the Department of Counselling Psychology at the University of British Columbia. She also runs her own private practice, Nexus Counselling Services, where she works as a psychotherapist clinical counsellor. Candace's developing expertise is focused on clients with post-traumatic stress, ritualistic abuse, dissociative disorders, and conflicts within interpersonal relationships. Candace was a research assistant, performer, and clinical therapist in the first production of *Contact!Unload* in April/May 2015.

Blair McLean holds an MA in counselling psychology from the University of British Columbia and is a Registered Clinical Counsellor with the BC Association of Clinical Counsellors. He was a videographer on the *Contact!Unload* project and has completed a film about the creation, rehearsal, and performance, which can be accessed through cIRcle on the UBC Library website. Blair works at Vancouver Community College as a counsellor.

Jennica Nichols is a PhD candidate in interdisciplinary studies at the University of British Columbia, with interests in intervention design, program evaluation, research-based theatre, and implementation science. She holds a Master of Public Health (Epidemiology, Global Health) degree from the University of Toronto (2012) and the Credentialed Evaluator designation from the Canadian Evaluation Society (2015).

John S. Ogrodniczuk is a professor of psychiatry and director of the Psychotherapy Program at the University of British Columbia. He has a particular interest in studying psychodynamic psychotherapy, personality disorders, group psychotherapy, alexithymia, and men's mental health. Dr. Ogrodniczuk has held several grants to support his research and has published extensively. He is the founder of HeadsUpGuys, an online resource that supports men in their fight against depression by providing tips, tools, information about professional services, and stories of success.

Marion Porath was professor emerita in the Department of Educational and Counselling Psychology, and Special Education at the University of British Columbia. She had a strong interest in arts-based ways of eliciting and telling personal stories of learning and development. Marion was the chair of the Gifted Program in the Faculty of Education for over two decades. Sadly, Dr. Porath passed away during the writing of this book.

JS Valdez's work is about listening deeply to the taken-for-grantedness of what it means to be present with Self and others. The lens with which Valdez listens, witnesses, and creates is shaped and informed by her roles as mother, wife, daughter, sister, immigrant-settler, and student in a doctoral program in Language and Literacy Education at the University of British Columbia, located on traditional, ancestral, and unceded land of the Musqueam peoples. JS was assistant director of the original creation process and production of *Contact!Unload* in 2015.

Marv Westwood is Professor Emeritus (Counselling Psychology Program) in the Department of Educational and Counselling Psychology, and Special Education at the University of British Columbia. He is recognized internationally for the development of the Veterans Transition Program (vtncanada.org), and is the co-project lead of *Contact!Unload.*

Index

Notes: "P" before a page number indicates script pages; italicized page numbers indicate a figure

Abandoned Brothers (play), 7, 17n19, 91
academic norms, 74, 76, 120
activation
    of audience members, 156–57, 161
    of civilian members, 12
    counselling support and, 12, 14, 39, 74–78, *75*, 161
    of veterans, 12, 39, 42, 48, 82, 85, 90
Afghanistan combat mission
    artworks honouring soldiers, 65–67;
        lestweforgetCANADA mural project,
        65–67, *66*, *67*, 157n1; SERIOUSshit art
        project, *69*, 124, *126*; Tribute Pole
    death statistics of soldiers and veterans,
        51, 128
    mental illness related to, 21. *See also*
        post-traumatic stress (PTS)
    soldiers' sense of purpose and, 71, 76,
        105
African child soldiers, 24
armed forces. *See* deaths of soldiers; military culture; suicide; veterans
arts
    role in deepening understanding, 75–76, 131, 151–52
    synergy between visual arts and theatre, 11
    See also artworks; poems; theatre
artworks
    IEDs, 65
    Illuminating the military experience
        (collage), *154*

    incorporating Canadian flag, 65
    as instruments for audience evaluation,
        166, 168, 172–75
    lestweforgetCANADA mural project,
        65–67, *66*, 157n1
    SERIOUSshit art project, *69*, 124,
        126
audience reactions, 78, 80, 118–19, 123–33,
    135–38, 151–57, 170–71
    formal evaluations of: integration into
        the theatre experience, 166, 168;
        interviews and focus groups, 40, 161–
        62, 166, 168–69; key findings, 162–65;
        limitations of, 169; participatory art
        installation, 166, 168, 172–75; post-
        performance surveys, 160–61, 162,
        166; pre-performance questions, 165–
        66; recommendations concerning,
        167–71
    role in therapeutic process, 43, 75, 85–
        86, 98–99, 119; mirroring of emo-
        tions, 40–41, 98–99; vicarious
        witnessing, 152–56, 176
    veterans, 4, 33, 37, 59–60
Australia
    Difficult Return research project, 22, 32–
        33, 91. *See also Return, The* (play)
    performances of *UNLOAD*, 70
    veterans' organizations, 23
authenticity
    role in recovery, 106–7, 111, 116–17
    in script, 59–60

Balfour, Michael, 7, 60, 91, 178
Banister, Elizabeth, 178
  personal experiences of play, 155–56
battle fatigue. *See* post-traumatic stress
  (PTS)
behavioural rehearsal, 28, 42, 43, 89
Belliveau, George, 178
  collaboration with *Difficult Return*
    research project, 22
  development of *Contact!Unload,* 10,
    11–12, 53–54, 59, 60
  in photographs, *P15, P61*
  roles, 112, 113–14, 120, *P15*
  views on therapeutic value, 98
Black Sedan (song), 124, 134*n*3
Blois, France, 144, 147*n*18, 147*n*19
Bokenfohr, Luke
  personal experiences of play, 79, 86
  in photographs, *5, P61*
British War Office Committee on Shell
  Shock, 27
Buchanan, Marla, 178
  personal experiences of play, 154–55

Campbell, Gordon, 5, 67
Canada House (London, Eng.), 4, 5
  lestweforgetCANADA mural, 67
  performance of *Contact!Unload,* 68
  Tribute Pole, 67–68
Canadian War Museum
  lestweforgetCANADA mural, 66–67
Cassel Hospital (Merseyside, Eng.), 27
catharsis, 14, 32–33, 40–41, 66, 85
  civilian participants, 90–91
cathartic witnessing, 98
ceremony, 30–31
civilian participants
  group cohesion and collaboration, 12,
    74–79, 113, 116
  impact of play on, 15, 89–91. *See also*
    audience reactions
Clews, Stephen
  collaboration with Foster Eastman,
    65, 67
  personal experience of play, 79
  in photographs, *5, P61*
Columbia
  veterans, 24
Combat Stress (organization), 22

Contact!Unload (play)
  community-university collaboration, 4,
    22, 54–55, 77, 149, 176–77
  companies: original production, 3–4,
    P6; touring productions, 70, *P6–P7*
  development process, 3–4, 10–16
  drama exercises, 113–14
  dramatis personae, *P2*
  group cohesion and collaboration:
    civilian members and, 12, 74–79,
    113, 116; creating trust and safety, 10,
    13, 39, 41, 55, 74–77, 98–99, 111–17;
    ingroup/outgroup identities, 109–10,
    119–20; veteran members and, 12, 41,
    86–88, 112–13, 115, 116
  music, 13, 118, 134*n*3, *P10*
  post-performance debriefings, 79–92,
    119, 156–57
  production timeline, 15–16
  program, 2015, *P3–P5*
  role of women in, 117–18, 121, 134*n*6,
    139–40, 170–71
  set, *P9–P10*
  support of Movember Canada, 3, 67,
    68, 171
  versions, 4; *UNLOAD,* 70
  veterans: motivation for participating,
    14–15, 37, 39–40, 57, 72, 80, 112
  See also audience reactions; performers
    in *Contact!Unload;* script of
    Contact!Unload; Tribute Pole
Cook, Christopher, 179
counselling support
  activation and, 12, 14, 39, 74–78, *75,*
    156–57, 161
  group counselling, 111–12; treatment of
    PTS, 97–98
Cox, Susan M., 179
Cry Havoc! (play), 6

deaths of soldiers
  effects on families, 129, 132–33, 134*n*3,
    P36–P39
  memorialized in artworks, 30–31, 65–
    69, 124, 126, 157*n*1
  See also suicide
DE-CRUIT (theatrical initiative), 6
Dennison, Britney, 179
depression (mental illness), 148–49

Difficult Return research project, 22, 32–33, 91
  See also Return, The (play)
Doerr, Anthony
  All the Light We Cannot See, 135, 136
Doerries, Bryan, 5
drama-based programs, 39
  behavioural rehearsal, 28, 42, 43, 89
  developmental transformations, 28–29
  embodiment, 82–85
  therapeutic value, 32, 38–43, 91–92
  See also research-based theatre; therapeutic enactment (TE)
dropping the baggage, 41, 50
Dry Hooch (organization), 23
Duff, Heather, 179
  poem by, 141–46

Eastman, Foster, 179–80
  artworks honouring soldiers, 65–67, *66*, *69*, 126, 157*n1*
  musician in *UNLOAD*, 70
  studio workspace, 11, 126
  See also Tribute Pole
embodied simulation, 40–41
embodied trauma, 81–84
embodiment, 82–83
  role of tableaux, 96–97
ethical concerns
  for audiences, 156–57
  inclusion of women, 140
  for participants, 91–92
  in writing of *Contact!Unload*, 55, 59–60

Fallujah (opera), 39
families
  effects of deaths of soldiers on, 129, 132–33, 134*n3*, P36–P39
  roles in veteran transition to civilian life, 120–21
family-sculpting techniques, 96
Feast of Crispian (theatrical initiative), 6–7
Fels, Lynn
  personal experience of play, 123–34
  poem by, 123
filmed version of *Contact!Unload* (play), 4
fire-team metaphor, 86–87

First World War
  treatment of PTS, 25–27, 38
Fisher, Gordon
  reflections on shell shock, 25–26

Garthside, Tim, 79, 180
  mental anguish, 3, 46–49, 52, 56, 105–7; treatment for PTS, 49–51, 105–8
  personal experiences as framework for play, 61, 62
  personal experiences of play, 77–79, 81–85, 107–8
  in photographs, *11, 14*, 62, *75*, P41
  poem by, P40–P41
  pre-play discussions, 56, 57, 61
gender
  male role socialization in military, 94–95, 109, 155
  post-traumatic stress and, 94–95
  relational-cultural theory and, 111
  See also masculine ideals; women
generative risk taking, 39, 75–78, 116, 118
Geraghty, Warren
  personal experiences of play, 79, 81
  photographs of, *5, 11, 14*, 79, P16, P34, P41, P61
  pre-play discussions, 56
Goddard, Nichola, 140
Gordon, Alistair G., 180
Greek drama
  representation of war, 5, 24, 38
grief, 10, 30–31
  families, 129, 132–33, 134*n3*, P36–P39
group counselling, 111–12
  in treatment of PTS, 97–98
guilt, 28, 38, 50–51, 85–86
  survivors' guilt, 10, 126–27, P25–P31

Hamilton, Dale
  band of brothers, 59, 77, 86, 130, P47
  collaboration with Foster Eastman, 67
  personal experiences of play, 79, 89
  in photographs, *11, 14*, P16, P34, P41, P47
  poem adapted from his writings, P33
  pre-play discussion, 59
Harry, Prince, Duke of Sussex, 4, *5*, 68
  comments on play, xiv
Hassall, Linda, 7, 13, 91

Henry V (William Shakespeare), 8
  as framework for *Contact!Unload*, 8, 13,
    54, 59, 61, P12, P14–P16, P24, P46
Hudspeth, Julie, 70
Hurst, Arthur, 26

Illuminating the military experience
    (collage), 154
Invictus Games, 2017, 68–69
irritable heart. *See* post-traumatic stress
    (PTS)

James, Miller, 28
Johnson, David Read, 28, 29–30

Keefe, Anna, 180
  grandfathers' war experiences, 73–74,
    76, 78
  personal experiences of play, 74–78
Kivari, Carson, *11*, 180–81
Kuhl, David
  performing role in play, 14
  role in Veterans Transition Program, 4

Laidler, Tim, 181
  collaboration with Foster Eastman, 65
  personal experiences, 71–72
Lea, Graham W., 181
  participant/observer role, 56–57
  personal trauma, 55, 56, 57
  stage management role, 53–54, 60, 61,
    62, 63, P8
  writing of *Contact!Unload*, 10, 12, 52;
    early challenges, 3, 53–60, 62–63;
    ethical concerns, 55, 59–60; shaping
    the script, 60–62
Leggo, Carl, 181
  memories of father-in-law, 135–37
  personal experience of play, 135–38
  poems by, 136–37
lestweforgetCANADA mural project, 65–
    67, *66*
  as part of *Contact!Unload*, 67, 157n1
Lewis, Jonathan, 7
Longman, Oliver, 89–90
  in photographs, *11*, *14*, *127*, *P34*
Lopresti, Phillip, 70, 181
  military experience, 94, 96, 181
  in photographs, *27*, *P34*

MacKinnon, Chuck, 132, 181
  mental anguish, 37
  personal experiences of play, 37, 79, 80,
    81, 88–89
  in photographs, *5*, *14*, *62*, *127*, *P16*, *P61*
  pre-play discussion, 60, 62–63
Malaal, Parween Faiz Zadah
  poem by, 139
Man/Art/Action project, 67
  See also Contact!Unload (play); Tribute
    Pole
Marshall, Candace, 182
  personal experiences of play, 114, 115,
    116, 117–18, 121
  in photographs, *11*, *14*, *P41*
  practitioner perspective, 110
  roles, 109, 117–18
masculine ideals
  alignment with theatrical performance,
    93, 95–96
  as barriers to treatment, 148–49
  emotional connection and, 111
  See also military culture
Mates for Mates (organization), 23
McLean, Blair, 98, 182
mental illness, 148–49
  related to Afghanistan mission, 21
  stigmatization, 21
  See also post-traumatic stress (PTS);
    suicide
military culture
  male gender role socialization, 94–95,
    109, 155
  physicality, 56, 96
  social connectedness, 86–88, 109
  women soldiers and, 95, 140
  See also masculine ideals
The Military Museums (Calgary), 68
military veterans. *See* veterans
Movember Canada
  support for *Contact!Unload* project, 3,
    67, 68, 171
Mulkey, Marty, 30
music in *Contact!Unload*, 13, 118, 134n3, P10

narrative therapy, 99
Nichols, Jennica, 98, 172–73, 182

Ochsendorf, Jon, 118, 134n3

O'Connor, Alison, 7
Ogrodniczuk, John, 182
    memories of grandfather, 148–49
O'Toole, Erin, xiii
Overton, Matthew, xii, 67

pension neurosis. *See* post-traumatic
    stress (PTS)
performers in *Contact!Unload*, 14
    civilians, 14, 15, 18*n*35, 73–79, 117–18
    lack of diversity among, 173
    veterans, 14, 18*n*35, 39, 71–72, 74, 117,
        118; catharsis and normalization, 14,
        32–33, 40–41, 85; improvement of
        relational resiliency, 114, 120–21; mo-
        tivation for participating, 14–15, 37,
        39–40, 57, 72, 80, 112; sense of self as
        role models, 14, 32–33. *See also*
        Bokenfohr, Luke; Clews, Stephen;
        Garthside, Tim; Geraghty, Warren;
        Hamilton, Dale; MacKinnon, Chuck
performing war
    defined, 151
play (dramatherapy), 30, 82
poems
    by Carl Leggo, 136–37
    by Heather Duff, 141–46
    by JS Valdez, 172–75
    by Lynn Fels, 123
    by Parween Faiz Zadah Malaal, 139
    within the play, 13; by Dale Hamilton,
        P33; by Tim Garthside, P40–P41
poet(h)ic inquiry, 146*n*2
Porath, Marion, 182
    personal experiences of play, 151, 153, *154*
post-traumatic stress (PTS)
    causes: sustained exposure to trauma,
        28; Tim Garthside's experience, 28,
        46–49, 107; transgressions against
        moral beliefs, 28, 50–51, 107
    complications: avoidance of therapy,
        95, 148–49; delayed/inadequate
        treatment, 21, 28, 48–49; mistrust of
        civilians, 88, 109, 112, 113; secondary
        trauma of return, 28, 71
    effects and symptoms, 25, 48, 97, 109;
        anger and irritability, xii, 25, 48,
        50, 95, 97, 109, 163, 170; emotional
        avoidance and disconnection, 25,

29, 43, 46, 71, 97, 106–7, 109, 111, 120;
    gender-related differences, 94–95;
    guilt, 28, 38, 50–51, 85–86; panic
    attacks, 48, 116; profound changes
    in identity, 21–22, 49, 88; survivors'
    guilt, 10, 126–27, P25–P31; on veter-
    ans' bodies, 39, 41, 97–98, 107
gender differences, 94–95
historical vocabulary, 24–25, 38
inadequate treatment, 21, 28, 48–49
incidence of, 21
non-combat PTS compared, 28
recognition of, 24–25, 38
reluctance to recognize officially, 25–
    26, 27
See also treatment of PTS
Prideaux, Francis, 27
PTSD. *See* post-traumatic stress (PTS)

Rayne, Stephen, 7
Rayneard, Max, 6
Re-enacting the Battle of Seale Hayne
    (film), 26, 34*n*23
relational-cultural theory (RCT), 110–11
    as framework for analyzing
        Contact!Unload project, 111–21
Re-Live (theatrical initiative), 7
"Remembering" (poem), 136–37
research data
    on audience reactions, 160–71
    on impact on veterans, 79–92
research-based theatre
    evaluation methodology, 169–70, 171*n*3
    See also Contact!Unload (play); *Return,
        The* (play)
Return, The (play), 7, 22, 33
    scenes adapted for *Contact!Unload*,
        13, 60
risk
    as generative, 39, 75–78, 116, 118
ritual, 30–31

script of *Contact!Unload*
    basic framework elements, 54, 55, 61;
        Chuck MacKinnon's story, 62–63;
        playwright's experiences, 61, 62–63;
        Six Characters in Search of an Author
        (play), 10, 54, 58, 59; St. Crispin's Day
        speech, 8, 13, 54, 59, 61, P12, P14–P16,

P24, P46; tableaux, 60; therapeutic enactment, 57, 61; Tim Garthside's story, 61, 62; Tribute Pole, 61–62
collaborative development, 54–60, 115; veteran participation, 3–4, 55–63, 115
incorporation of poems & songs, 13, P33, P40–P41
incorporation of therapeutic enactment, 8, 13, 39, 57, P50–P59
use of soldiers' language, 41, 56
See also Contact!Unload (play)
Seale Hayne Hospital (England), 26, 34n23
Second World War
All the Light We Cannot See, 135, 136
experiences of family members, 73–74, 135–36, 137
treatment of PTS, 27, 38
secondary trauma of return, 28
SERIOUSshit art project, 69, 124, 126
Shakespearean texts
in Contact!Unload, 8, 10; St. Crispin's Day speech, 8, 13, 54, 59, 61, P12, P14–P16, P24, P46
role in theatrical initiatives, 6–7
Sheers, Owen, 7
shell shock. See post-traumatic stress (PTS)
Shell Shock (play), 39
Six Characters in Search of an Author (play)
as framework for Contact!Unload, 10, 54, 58, 59
Soldier On (play), 7
Soldiers' Arts Academy, 7
soldier's heart. See post-traumatic stress (PTS)
stage management, 10
Stand Tall (organization), 23
stigmatization
mental health issues and, 21
"Still Remembering" (poem), 137–38
suicide
incidence among men in general, 149
incidence among veterans: Canada, 51, 128; United States, 4, 6, 51
PTS and, 128–29, 130
SERIOUSshit art project, 69, 124, 126
See also deaths of soldiers
survivors' guilt, 10, 126–27, P25–P31

tableaux, 60
photographs of, 11, 127
therapeutic value, 12, 96–97, 99
The Telling Project (theatrical initiative), 6
theatre
role in facilitating transition to civilian life, 5–8
See also drama-based programs; research-based theatre; therapeutic enactment (TE)
therapeutic enactment (TE), 4, 7, 9, 39, 42–43
behavioural rehearsal, 42
five phases of, 9
motivation for sharing personal stories, 51
role in Contact!Unload, 4, 8, 11–12, 13, 39, 40–43, 42, 57, P50–P59
role in Veterans Transition Program (VTP), 8–10, 32–33, 50–51
"Tomb, the Unknown Soldier's Wife" (poem), 141–46
trauma, 28, 38
embodied, 39, 41, 42, 81–84
Tim Garthside's experience, 46–48, 81–82
See also post-traumatic stress (PTS); treatment of PTS
treatment of PTS
arts and health practices, 22–24, 28–33; embodied process, 95–97; group identity, 109–10; role of ceremonies and ritual, 30–31; role of play in, 30; Vietnam War and, 28. See also artworks; drama-based programs; research-based theatre; therapeutic enactment (TE)
First and Second Generation programs, 29
group counselling, 97–98
historical shifts, 25–27, 28–31, 38–39
Tim Garthside's experiences, 49–52
Tribute Pole
audience reaction to, 124–25
carving of, 11, 67
role in Contact!Unload, 11, 13, 61–62, 67–68, P9–P10; raising of Pole, 14, 124, P10
symbolism of, 67

Tricomi, Lisa, 6
triggering. *See* activation
True Patriot Love Foundation, 66
The Two Worlds of Charlie F. (play), 7

Under the Wire (theatre company), 5
United Kingdom, 22
　World War I treatment of PTS, 25–27
United States
　National Initiative for Arts and Health
　　in the Military, 22, 23
　post-World War I treatment of PTS, 27
　veterans' organizations, 23
　Vietnam Veterans Memorial (Washing-
　　ton, DC), 30–31
　Vietnam War veterans, 28–31, 38–39
University of British Columbia, 54–55, 77,
　92n1, 149
　Veterans Transition Program, xiii, 4,
　8, 22
the unknown soldier, 141
UNLOAD (play), 70

Valdez, JS, *14, 75,* 82, 117, 174–75, 183
　poem by, 173–74
veterans
　bonds with each other, 117, 135–36
　difficulties in transition to civilian life:
　　key themes, 10, 54; mental health
　　issues, 3, 21–22, 109; mistrust of civil-
　　ians, 88, 109, 112–13
　mental health difficulties, 3, 4, 21
　motivation for participating, 14–15, 37,
　　39–40, 57, 72, 80, 112
　women, 140
　See also Bokenfohr, Luke; Clews,
　　Stephen; Garthside, Tim; Geraghty,
　　Warren; Hamilton, Dale;
　　MacKinnon, Chuck; performers
　　in *Contact!Unload;* post-traumatic
　　stress (PTS)
Veterans Affairs Canada, 48–49, 140
Veterans and Families Institute for
　Military Social Research, 22

veterans' organizations, 23
Veterans Transition Network (VTN), xiii,
　18n36, 43
Veterans Transition Program (VTP), 4, 8,
　18n36, 22, 50
　dropping baggage, 41, 50
　role of therapeutic enactment in, 8–10,
　　32–33, 50–51
　Tim Garthside's experiences, 49–52
vicarious witnessing, 151–57
Vietnam Veterans Memorial (Washington,
　DC), 30–31
Vietnam War veterans, 28–31, 38–39
visual art. *See* artworks

war and aftermath
　representation in literature and theatre,
　　5, 24, 38
war neurosis. *See* post-traumatic stress
　(PTS)
Waterman, Mike, 90–91
　in photographs, *5, 11, P15, P47, P61*
Wei, Jonathan, 6
Westwood, Marv, *5, 11,* 43, 183
　collaboration with Australian project,
　　22
　development of play, 10–16, 54, 57, 120
　roles, 14, *75,* 79, 91, 112, *P16*
　Veterans Transition Program, 4, 49
Wilkinson, Linden, 70
Wolfert, Stephan, 6
women
　experience of war, 134n6, 139–46
　military culture and, 95, 140
　roles in *Contact!Unload,* 117–18, 121,
　　134n6, 139–40, 170–71
　roles in veteran transition, 120–21
　veterans, 140

Xwalacktun
　carving of Tribute Pole, 67

Young Diggers (organization), 23

STUDIES IN CANADIAN MILITARY HISTORY

John Griffith Armstrong, *The Halifax Explosion and the Royal Canadian Navy: Inquiry and Intrigue*

Andrew Richter, *Avoiding Armageddon: Canadian Military Strategy and Nuclear Weapons, 1950-63*

William Johnston, *A War of Patrols: Canadian Army Operations in Korea*

Julian Gwyn, *Frigates and Foremasts: The North American Squadron in Nova Scotia Waters, 1745-1815*

Jeffrey A. Keshen, *Saints, Sinners, and Soldiers: Canada's Second World War*

Desmond Morton, *Fight or Pay: Soldiers' Families in the Great War*

Douglas E. Delaney, *The Soldiers' General: Bert Hoffmeister at War*

Michael Whitby, ed., *Commanding Canadians: The Second World War Diaries of A.F.C. Layard*

Martin F. Auger, *Prisoners of the Home Front: German POWs and "Enemy Aliens" in Southern Quebec, 1940-46*

Tim Cook, *Clio's Warriors: Canadian Historians and the Writing of the World Wars*

Serge Marc Durflinger, *Fighting from Home: The Second World War in Verdun, Quebec*

Richard O. Mayne, *Betrayed: Scandal, Politics, and Canadian Naval Leadership*

P. Whitney Lackenbauer, *Battle Grounds: The Canadian Military and Aboriginal Lands*

Cynthia Toman, *An Officer and a Lady: Canadian Military Nursing and the Second World War*

Michael Petrou, *Renegades: Canadians in the Spanish Civil War*

Amy J. Shaw, *Crisis of Conscience: Conscientious Objection in Canada during the First World War*

Serge Marc Durflinger, *Veterans with a Vision: Canada's War Blinded in Peace and War*

James G. Fergusson, *Canada and Ballistic Missile Defence, 1954-2009: Déjà Vu All Over Again*

Benjamin Isitt, *From Victoria to Vladivostok: Canada's Siberian Expedition, 1917-19*

James Wood, *Militia Myths: Ideas of the Canadian Citizen Soldier, 1896-1921*

Timothy Balzer, *The Information Front: The Canadian Army and News Management during the Second World War*

Andrew B. Godefroy, *Defence and Discovery: Canada's Military Space Program, 1945-74*

Douglas E. Delaney, *Corps Commanders: Five British and Canadian Generals at War, 1939-45*

Timothy Wilford, *Canada's Road to the Pacific War: Intelligence, Strategy, and the Far East Crisis*

Randall Wakelam, *Cold War Fighters: Canadian Aircraft Procurement, 1945-54*

Andrew Burtch, *Give Me Shelter: The Failure of Canada's Cold War Civil Defence*

Wendy Cuthbertson, *Labour Goes to War: The CIO and the Construction of a New Social Order, 1939-45*

P. Whitney Lackenbauer, *The Canadian Rangers: A Living History*

Teresa Iacobelli, *Death or Deliverance: Canadian Courts Martial in the Great War*

Graham Broad, *A Small Price to Pay: Consumer Culture on the Canadian Home Front, 1939-45*

Peter Kasurak, *A National Force: The Evolution of Canada's Army, 1950-2000*

Isabel Campbell, *Unlikely Diplomats: The Canadian Brigade in Germany, 1951-64*

Richard M. Reid, *African Canadians in Union Blue: Volunteering for the Cause in the Civil War*

Andrew B. Godefroy, *In Peace Prepared: Innovation and Adaptation in Canada's Cold War Army*

Nic Clarke, *Unwanted Warriors: The Rejected Volunteers of the Canadian Expeditionary Force*

David Zimmerman, *Maritime Command Pacific: The Royal Canadian Navy's West Coast Fleet in the Early Cold War*

Cynthia Toman, *Sister Soldiers of the Great War: The Nurses of the Canadian Army Medical Corps*

Daniel Byers, *Zombie Army: The Canadian Army and Conscription in the Second World War*

J.L. Granatstein, *The Weight of Command: Voices of Canada's Second World War Generals and Those Who Knew Them*

Colin McCullough, *Creating Canada's Peacekeeping Past*

Douglas E. Delaney and Serge Marc Durflinger, eds., *Capturing Hill 70: Canada's Forgotten Battle of the First World War*

Brandon R. Dimmel, *Engaging the Line: How the Great War Shaped the Canada–US Border*

Meghan Fitzpatrick, *Invisible Scars: Mental Trauma and the Korean War*

Patrick M. Dennis, *Reluctant Warriors: Canadian Conscripts and the Great War*

Frank Maas, *The Price of Alliance: The Politics and Procurement of Leopard Tanks for Canada's NATO Brigade*

Geoffrey Hayes, *Crerar's Lieutenants: Inventing the Canadian Junior Army Officer, 1939–45*

Richard Goette, *Sovereignty and Command in Canada–US Continental Air Defence, 1940–57*

Geoff Jackson, *The Empire on the Western Front: The British 62nd and Canadian 4th Divisions in Battle*

Steve Marti and William John Pratt, eds., *Fighting with the Empire: Canada, Britain, and Global Conflict, 1867–1947*

Steve Marti, *For Home and Empire: Voluntary Mobilization in Australia, Canada, and New Zealand during the First World War*

Peter Kasurak, *Canada's Mechanized Infantry: The Evolution of a Combat Arm, 1920–2012*

STUDIES IN CANADIAN MILITARY HISTORY
Published by UBC Press in association with the Canadian War Museum